The spoof guide to good practice on

How to do DRUGS

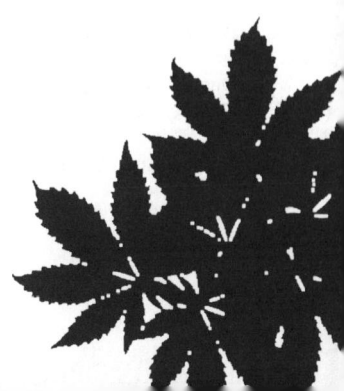

First published in Great Britain in 2005 by
Artnik
341b Queenstown Road
London SW8 4LH
UK

© **Artnik 2005**

All rights reserved. No part of this publication may be reproduced, stored in or introduced into a retrieval system, or transmitted in any form or by any means (electronic, mechanical, photocopying, recording or otherwise) without the prior written permission of both the copyright owner and the publisher of this book.

ISBN 1 903906 44 X

Design: Supriya Sahai
Editor: John McVicar

Printed and bound in Spain by Gráfica Diaz

The spoof guide to good practice on
How to do DRUGS

Charlie E. Crackhead

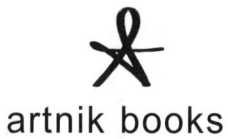

artnik books

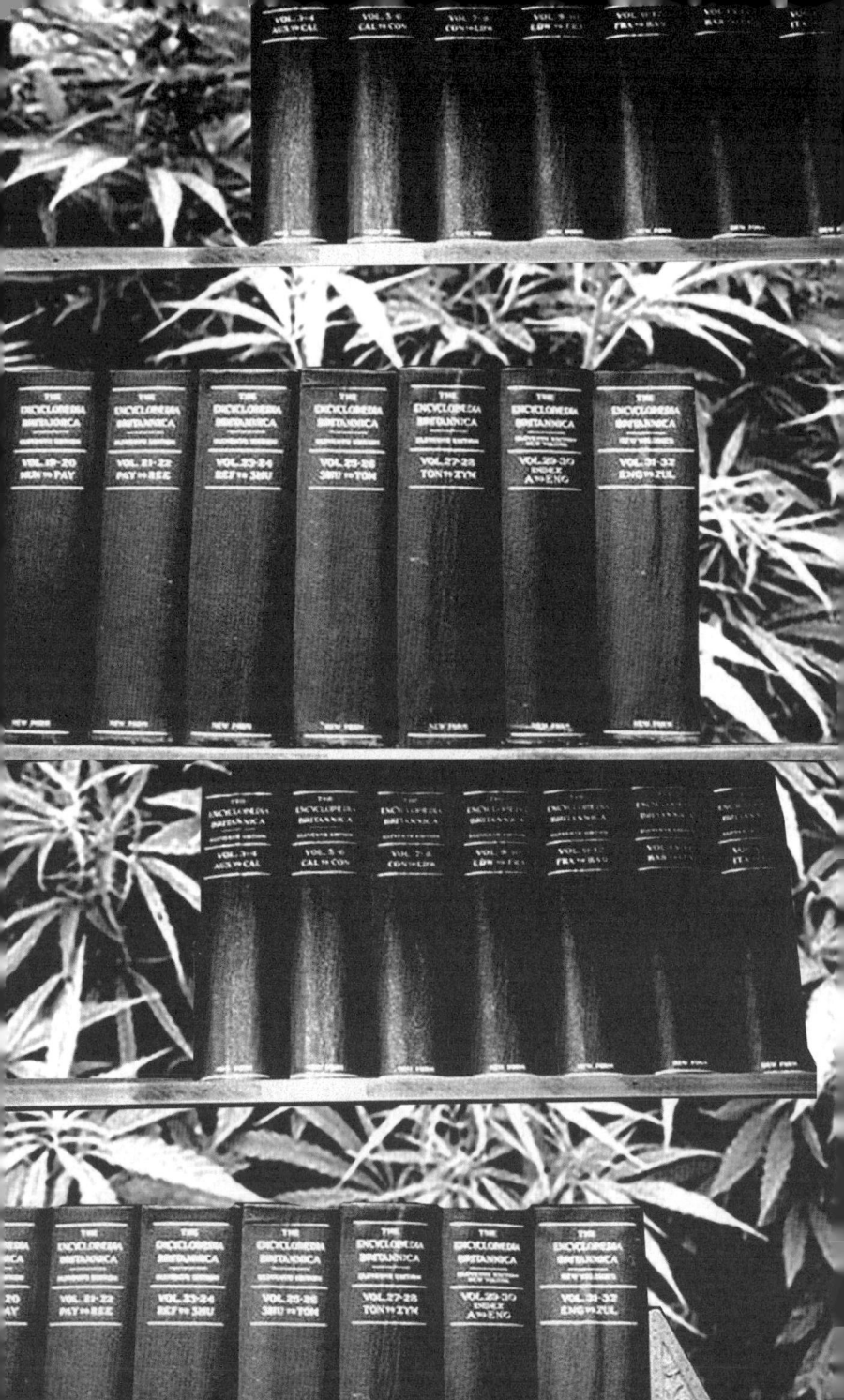

How to do Drugs

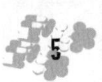

Rule Britannia

On the subject of drug addiction, the (now-discredited) 1930 Edition of Encyclopaedia Britannica divides addicts into two groups: the 'unfortunate' and the 'vicious'. The 'unfortunate' can be defined as good, middle-class people such as you or I, who are addicted only by mistake.

We do not succumb to the 'base and bestial intemperances of the low order'. No, we merely grow 'habitually accustomed' to the 'strong medicinal properties' contained in these substances; substances we might ingest to overcome 'legitimate natural ills' such as depression, boredom or having too much money.

> This misfortune should not be confused with criminality.

Very often a decent chap can become locked in a self-destructive pattern because of the sad fact of having more money than sense, a condition for which drugs are a proven cure. The situation can be exacerbated in the very rich by the lack of a need for gainful employment. These people deserve only our sympathy.

The true villains, the so-called 'vicious' group, are unemployed not

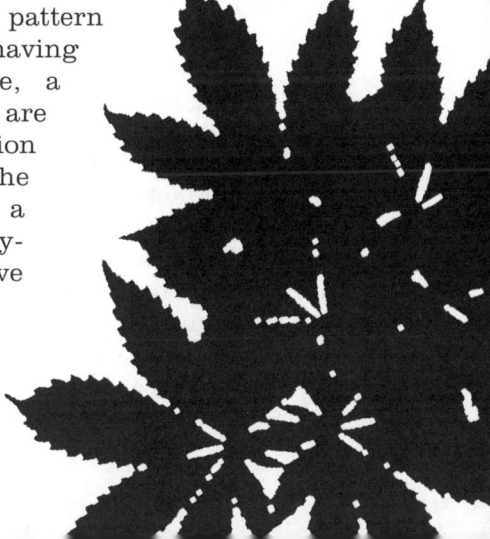

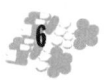

because they can afford to be, but because they know no better. In rare cases they may actually want a job but be incapable of securing one through lack of a decent education, or even a decent tie.

They have no money to speak of and STILL choose to spend what little they have on expensive luxuries like cocaine or heroin, and as such warrant no sympathy at all. It is the same working class 'false economy' that makes them buy the latest 'satellite dish' to pump 24-hour garbage into their grotty and ill-furnished council houses (or 'crack dens').

> The Encyclopaedia describes this class of addict as **'those that might be termed the vicious group, lacking in religion, motivation or moral fibre.'**

However, it points out that it is not known whether it is the drugs themselves that bring out these desperate qualities, or rather whether it is only those of fundamentally bad character who stray in the first place.

The author implies that a genetic blight, such as being working-class, demands a genetic solution. In this sense drugs could be seen as a society's gift to weed out those of undesirable stock. Perhaps these views are no longer fashionable; but before we judge our forefathers too harshly, remember that this kind of thinking dates from back in the 1930s, before 'Hitler' became a dirty word.

> The Enc Brit notes with relief that 'thankfully there are very few proper addicts in this country, and those that are generally collect in the Greater London area.'

It is also worth bearing in mind, however, that the compilers of this venerable fount of knowledge were not comfortable travelling north of Watford, and had probably never heard of Liverpool.

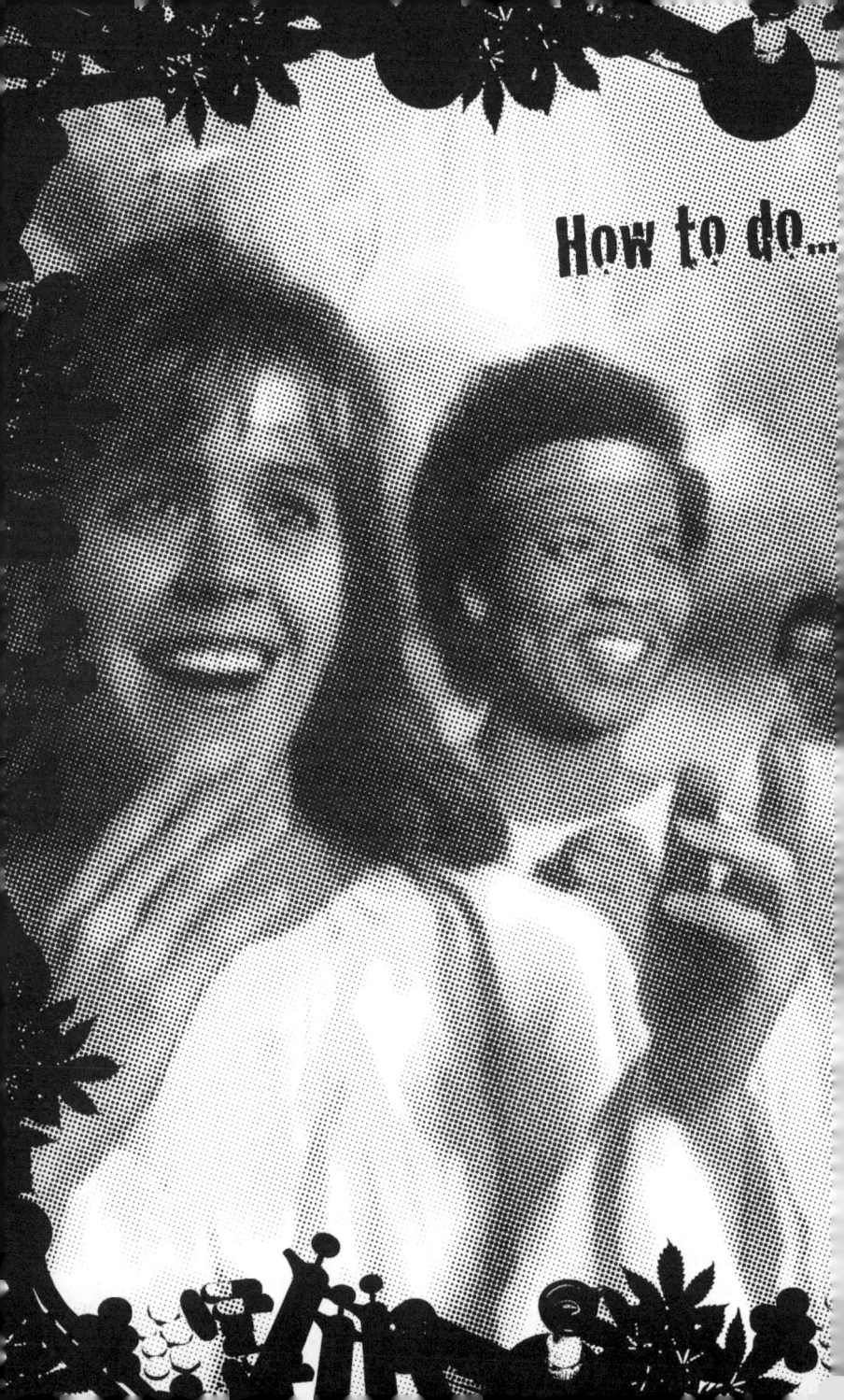

Contents

Introduction: Rule Brittania......................5
A Short Untrue History of Drugs......................12

How to take **Heroin**......................17
How to take **Cocaine**......................23
How to take **Crack**......................29
How to take **Speed**......................33
How to take **Ecstacy**......................37
How to take **Marijuana**......................47
Hallucigenics......................54
Paraphernalia......................58

Smuggling......................61
Where to find drugs and How to score......................67
    Social scoring
    Street scoring
    Scoring off tramps
        Scoring in a foreign country
        Scoring by mail-order
        Drug tour of Glasgow

Drugs in **Sports**......................87
Drugs and **Driving**......................93
Drugs and **Dining**......................101
Sex and Drugs......................105
Notes for **Parents**......................112
These are **NOT** drugs......................116
Celebrities and drugs......................120
Drugs and **Animals**......................122
Drugs and **Taxes**......................123
Drug **Talk**......................124

How to take **Drugs without Paying** for them......................127

How to take Drugs...

Introduction

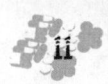

Books and leaflets on drug misuse are commonplace. Few, however, live up to their promise and actually advise you how to improve the way you use drugs. Follow these simple tips on how to maximise the pleasure and efficiency of your drug-taking and soon misuse of precious and expensive drugs will be a thing of the past.

This book is not intended as an endorsement of taking drugs. This book is not intended as a cautionary tale against taking drugs.

> This book works on the understanding that **drugs are a mundane reality; just another everyday pursuit, like sex or cooking,** that most people need help to do properly.

In turn this will hopefully be a happy reminder of why we all started in the first place.

This book will spice up your drug life, and perhaps even save your ailing marriage to narcotics.

In short, this is a simple guide to what makes it fun, and what makes it entirely painful to take drugs of all kinds, and how to make the most out of them while the fun lasts. Or you do.

Whichever is the longer.

Happy gurning.

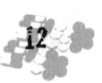

A Short Untrue History of DRUGS

The word 'drugs' comes from the Greek drogos, meaning 'happy time'. 'Narcotic' comes from two words, Narcos, meaning heavenly, and Tikka, meaning chicken.

This is because the first recreational drugs to be concocted in the land of philosophers were made from chickens.

Dried and smoked, the feathers were believed to help the user understand the future: a 'fowl-smelling oracle of Hades,' according to Herodotus, who used to trip out regularly on bags of rooster.

He describes lost afternoons spent lying on his back on the acropolis staring at the clouds, when he and his philosopher mates would bore passers-by with facile 'revelations' about dreams, space travel and the slender line between the tangible and the aesthetic.

However, it is believed that the search for a chemical high predates the science of Ancient Greeks. Neanderthals would snort ground-up mammoth-tusk as a coming-of-age ceremony, according to cave paintings found in Wigan.

They apparently depict some kind of prehistoric 'hunt ball', full of brash young warriors with bleeding noses gesticulating wildly and laughing at poor people.

The Egyptian pharaoh Tunfukt is believed to have commissioned the Sphinx based on a childish sketch he drew of a creature he

How to do Drugs

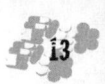

claimed was 'chasing him' whilst chewing on strange reeds – although it was more likely that the strong active ingredients made him confuse his wife and his cat.

(Later, these herbs were renamed 'khat' for this very reason – and contrary to widespread belief it is this kind of khat that they held sacred).

The bar was raised by the Romans, whose decadence knew no bounds. Young beavers and stoats were crushed and served on vine leaves for their pagan love-juices, as a form of primitive Viagra. Emperor Nero, in his memoirs, recalls an evening at an orgy tarnished by brewer's droop, eventually going to bed angry and alone after drinking three vials of liquid dormouse and oyster sweat.

When he woke up at midday he suddenly had such raging horn he couldn't get his toga on, charging back into the dining hall only to discover all the slave-girls had been executed, on his orders, in a frustrated late-night act of petulance.

Despite the uncultured reputation of the Vikings, many drugs that we still use today were first introduced to these shores by longboat. The earliest raiders were not the Danes or Norsemen, but sailors from the Low Countries.

The Vikings of Holland were more laid-back

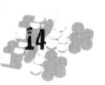

than their Northern cousins, less hooked on raping and pillaging and more into paying our womenfolk to dance on tables whilst inhaling thick dark smoke from earthenware pots.

This is perhaps why their invasions petered out and were superseded by the more aggressive tactics of the northern beserkers, fired-up on a combination of speed, sugary alcopops and shit music.

It seems the native Anglos were highly receptive to this vulgar and thuggish lifestyle, which eventually led to the foundation of many wine-bars along the East Coast now frequented by footballers.

With the spoilsport influence of the church, it would be centuries before the practice was revived in Europe.

As the Renaissance took hold, entrepreneurs and explorers – the likes of Columbus, Sir Francis Drake and Maris Piper – would import various roots and tubers from the Americas, then secretly hawk their exotic-looking wares down Cheapside in exchange for hand relief from sailors.

But the psychotropic effects were unspectacular; ironic, since the poppy was also being imported purely as an ornamental plant.

As our empire expanded, so did the

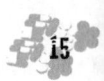

availability of drugs in Britain. Opium dens, as frequented by Victorian gentlemen of disrepute, are documented in the works of Wilde – but justly less famous were the glue dens of Bedlam.

Cheap and nasty, they were the domain of madmen and vicars who would squat around old warehouses with their cassocks over their heads until they got spots around their mouths.

> Poets have famously paid tribute to psychotropics; Coleridge's dreamlike poem 'Kola Khan' sung of 'sweet Venezuelan coco leaf/ dear powder of the Incan kings' (the critic Professor John Carey suggests a clever double meaning in the word 'dear').
> The poet was held in disgrace at the time, but the great and good of society have come to agree with his central thesis: COCAINE IS INDEED EXPENSIVE, AND ALL THE BETTER FOR IT.

So we have evolved a long way since the dubious recreational habits of the Greeks. But interestingly, the mind-altering qualities contained in parts of chickens – feathers, beak and legs – are still marketed to this very day.

Note the hyperactivity, visual disturbance and short-lived rush brought on by any visit to a KFC restaurant.

Afterwards, there are the headaches, the sweats and the spots around the mouth.

Perhaps the ancients have more to teach us than we like to admit.

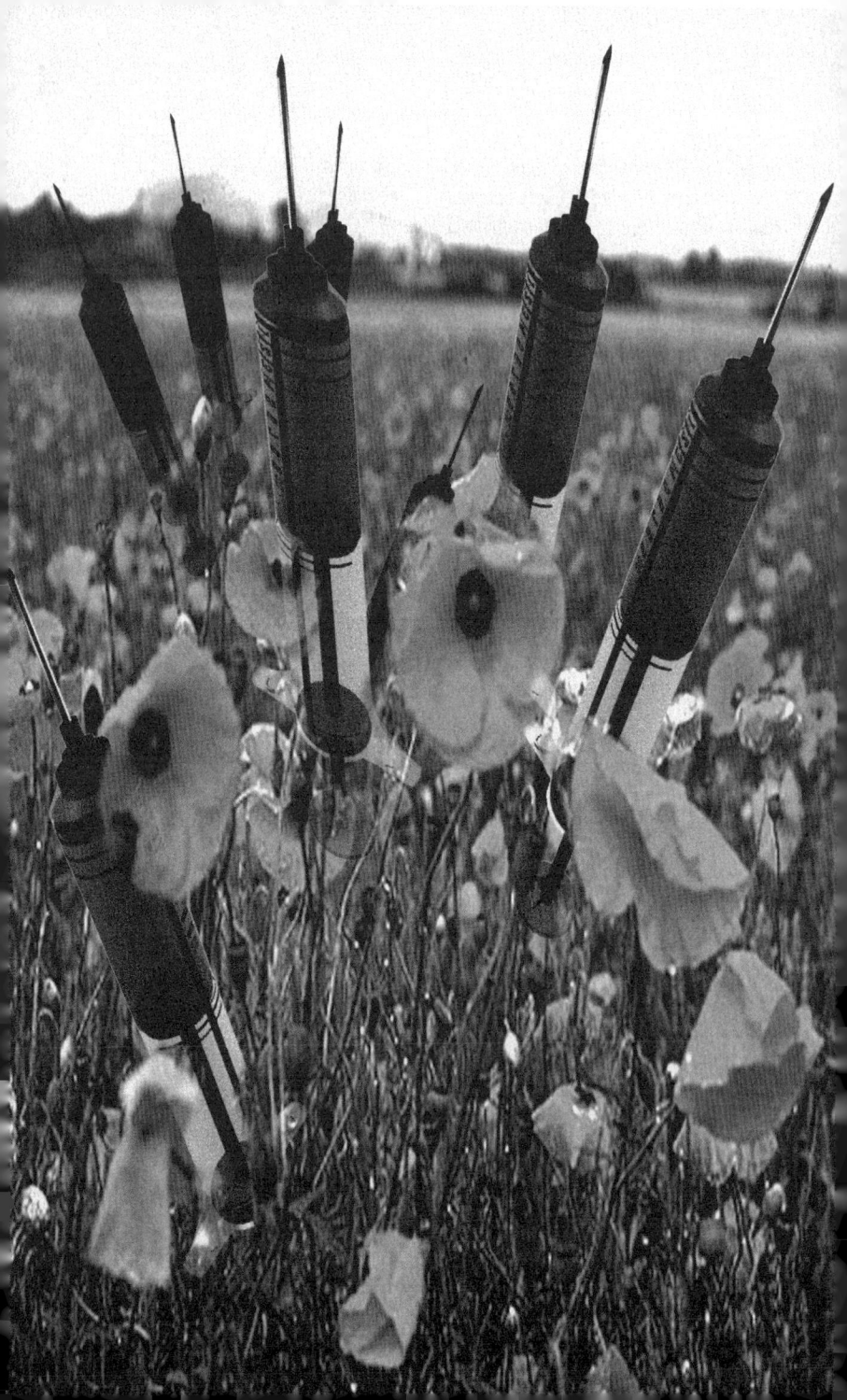

All your life you're taught that if something is white, it must be worse for you than something that is brown. Brown bread, brown rice, brown sugar; all healthier than their synthetic white cousins.

And all this received wisdom goes out of the window when you come to heroin. The upgrade from snow white to golden brown is definitely not a health kick.

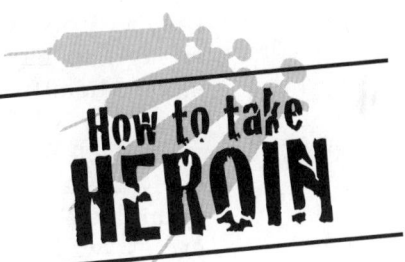

H is the the big one... perhaps the first chapter you might skip if a wet-behind-the-ears student, and the first page you'll turn to if an outraged tabloid editor.

The word heroin sounds to some just like one big dirty needle. **Actually, heroin comes in many forms.**

There is scag, which comes from tramps. There is opium, a more well-heeled, culturally refined form which Karl Marx memorably described as 'the religion of the masses' (he is often misquoted on this count).

And then there's the methadone, the morphine, the acetylcodeine, the compounds and cousins and derivatives, and all the ways and means enjoyed by thousands engaged in the half-hearted effort to kick the stuff.

A moral relativist might describe these forms as (respectively) bad, good and neutral.

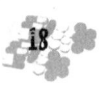

The medicinal ones are easy enough to deal with. They come in easy-to-swallow capsules or occasionally liquid form. They even come with instructions on the labels.

If you even have them in your possession then chances are you won't need telling what they're for: you must've been streetwise enough to have requested them by name or stolen them from an old folks' home.

In fact most civilians will ingest related derivatives every week in Lemsip Max and Feminax. You might be cursing junkies on the street while still relying on your own government-sanctioned dosages, using them to increase productivity at work rather than just keeping warm on the pavement.

Point this out to the flu-ridden desk-jockey beside you and it will most likely reinforce his unshakeable belief that the unemployed deadbeat junkie isn't a special case, he's just plain lazy. And he's probably right.

Opium is different.
THE UNITED NATIONS OFFICE ON DRUGS AND CRIME
defines opium as 'the coagulated juice from the unripe capsule of the poppy plant'.
What they don't say (but they should) is that an alternative definition would be 'a little taste of heaven in a straw.'

Why stop there? Once we admit that it's the greatest thing since sliced brown, we're away. Call it 'smoky plumes of blissful sepia, a

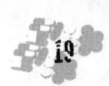

whispered cloud of angels breaking from feet of clay to dance on thin air' if you prefer. But you don't have to be lying in a Vietnamese bamboo hut or reclining in a notorious Victorian opium den to appreciate this experience fully.

Heaven can be purchased in foil for £10 a time and taken in the privacy of a street corner, or enjoyed with friends at the end of a hard day's capitalism.

Just buy a wrap of regular brown and line it up in the crease of some tin foil. Keep a rolled note or plastic straw in the mouth, with one hand holding the foil stiff and another running the lighter back and forth an inch or two under the surface: hey presto.

Your troubles will slip from your mind like they never existed, as you suck excitedly on the tube to make sure no curls of smoke escape your throat.

You will realise that all your life you've just been out in the cold collecting firewood and suddenly, wonderfully, you've come inside to the hearth and there's hot soup on the hob.

The only slight downside to this revelation is the after-effect: spending the rest of your life newly aware of how very chilly it is in the real world. Therefore the best way to experience this extreme philosophical truth without it ruining your life forever is: make sure you can't get hold of any more.

Lock the doors and burn your phonebook.

Before you take that first hit check you don't have enough left for a second. See that you have no more money or gear or means of obtaining it that evening.

Be a man and stop licking that coagulated sap that's left in the fold of your Kit-Kat wrapper. Understand that you can never experience a feeling quite like it again, so just let go and give up trying. Easy.

SOME COMMON MYTHS

So, now we've nailed the myth that heroin is very addictive – well, in the words of Harry Hill, maybe just a little moreish – it's time to look at some other myths involved with the substance.

> One, largely perpetuated by a grisly scene in Pulp Fiction, is that snorting a line of heroin is tantamount to putting a bullet in the head.

Well, it does feel a bit like that, largely because it is usually done by mistake, but depending on the size of the line it's perfectly possible to survive, even without the aid of an adrenaline shot through the ribcage.

In fact some find it a refreshingly direct way to enjoy the medicinal benefits offered by heroin. But do be careful, and make sure the floor beneath you is soft for the fall.

> Myth two is that if you inject a bubble of air into your veins it'll run to your heart and stop it dead.

Erm... and do you remember the other playground story, the one about chewing gum? 'If you accidentally swallow it then it sticks to your insides and kills you.' That's true also.

And my cousin's boyfriend's sister, she had this spider bite and it got bigger and bigger and grosser and grosser and then one day she went to a doctor and he burst it and a million baby spiders came out and crawled all over her.

Honestly, this one must be true as a doctor told me.

Needles are tricky little implements when rusty – and junkies are crude craftsmen, as often as not in no state to operate delicate machinery.

So the 'air bubble' scenario should be an everyday occurrence, but you still don't hear of too many people dying through this apparently simple act of carelessness. Even tired nurses would then be culpable on a regular basis.

As the great smackhead William Burroughs said, **if the story were true then there wouldn't be a junkie alive in America today.**

Mind you, just about everyone he was writing about has since died, so what the hell does he know?

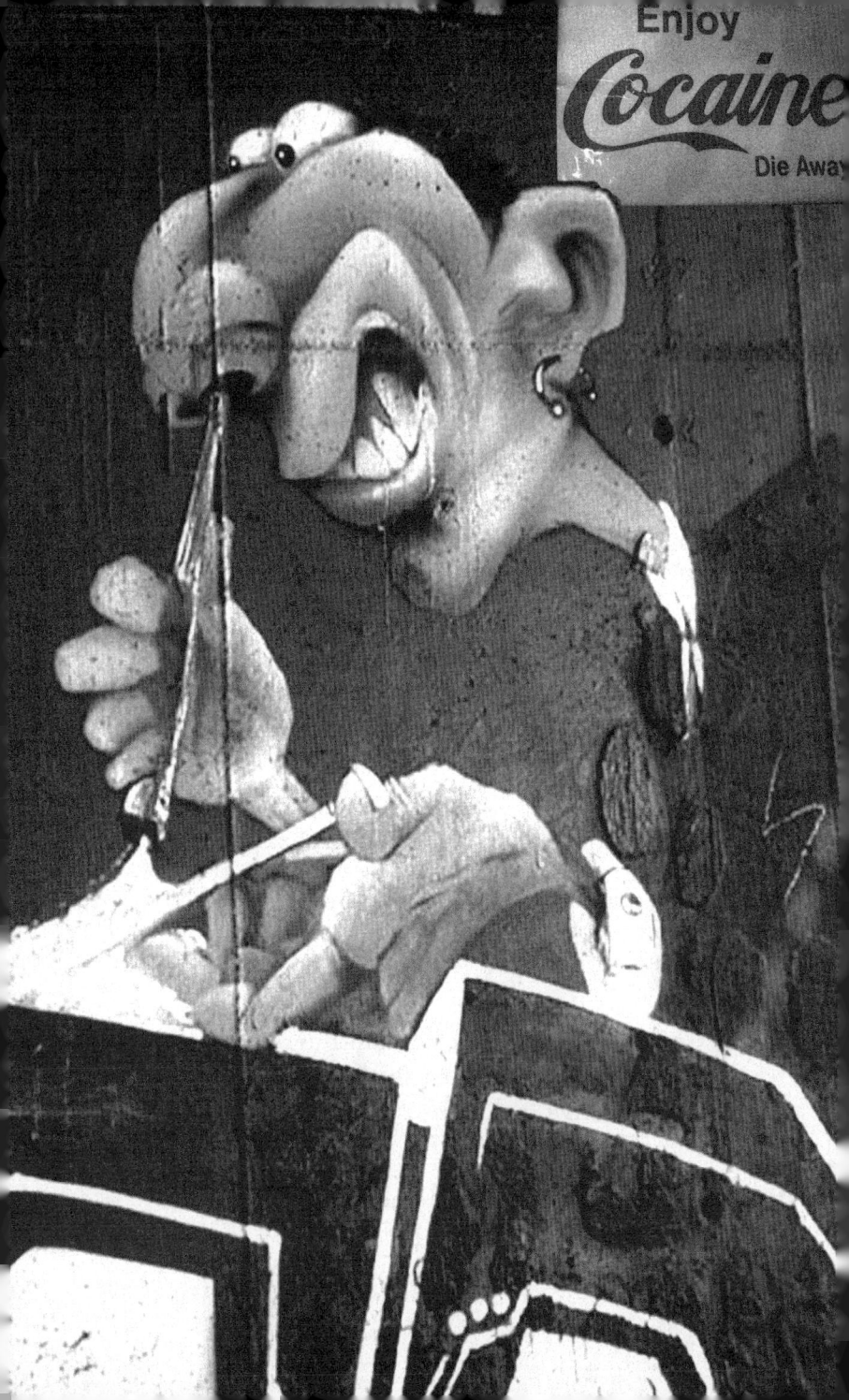

Increasingly, knowing how to take cocaine has evolved from an exotic and mysterious ritual to an entry-level necessity for anyone who wants to mix with the best society has to offer: idle rich, aristocracy, footballers, ad execs, **Sun** journalists, glamour models, reality TV stars, basically the top fifty percent. Oh, plus the bottom fifty percent whenever they can afford it.

How to take COCAINE

> TOP TIP: Don't use a golden straw and plated wallet except as a semi-ironic affectation among your very best friends. If you show such things off in front of casual acquaintances they will instinctively mistrust you. **They will believe you have something to prove – which, let's face it, you do.**

HOW TO ROLL A NOTE

A £50 note is just as ostentatious to produce at a party as a plated gold straw (and probably worth more, whatever the guy who produced it would have you believe).

However, it is more acceptable in polite drug etiquette, having as it does an established place in coke culture and history. A disadvantage is its greater length compared to smaller denominations, requiring a more sustained and powerful inhalation.

This only really becomes a problem as the evening progresses and sinuses begin to clog up, while basic co-ordination goes down the pan.

For this reason treat your 'fiddy' note like the very best champagne when the neighbours come round for Christmas drinks – something you wheel out at the beginning purely for effect, then withdraw discreetly and replace with cheaper stuff as the evening wears on.

Palates will become less discerning, and additionally you protect yourself against the light-fingeredness of houseguests who may try on the 'oh terribly sorry, I was sure it was mine' school of cash-pocketry (this rule of thumb also applies when you invite those slightly pikey neighbours round at Xmas).

Remember, they may not be bad people, just genuinely confused (moral sense is one of the first qualities to be affected by high-fidelity cocaine).

Even if you do get your money's worth back, chances are it'll have some stranger's blood down one end.

A £10, by comparison, is too common, and will get mixed up with everyone else's around the table.

A purpley one (£20) is therefore the best compromise of size, worth and class: perfect for everyday use.

A fiver is just too tiddly and cheap for public use; save it for when finding yourself, say, in the facilities of a public house on your own the next day.

It will be well suited to the skanky business of draining the lumpy dregs from the corner of a wrap. Its shorter size means you can hang it from one nostril and unfold the wrap in your hands, saving the bother of racking up on the loo-seat.

Remember, the additional time spent racking up in the bogs may lead gannet-like friends to work out you still have some left, which is clearly a total no-no.

Mind you, by this point a rolled-up tube ticket or grimy old receipt will do just as well.

> Cocaine is defined as 'one of a series of alkaloids occurring in the leaves of coca, a shrub indigenous to Bolivia and Peru, but now chiefly produced by cultivation in Java'
>
> (or so my 1930 Encyclopaedia would have you believe).
>
> (SOURCE: ENCYCLOPAEDIA BRITANNICA 1930, NOW THANKFULLY EX-COPYRIGHT)

Its geography may have become pandemic since then but the chemistry remains the same. Information you might like to know:

'Cocaine crystallises from alcohol in colourless prisms', which may explain those stomach aches during long nights on the razz.

'It melts at 98 degrees', explaining why all your efforts to turn it into home-made crack in the frying pan are doomed to messy failure.

'It is readily soluble in ordinary solvents except water' (but sad experience will tell you that water is the mortal enemy of a dry wrap, especially when falling into lavatory pans).

What do we learn from these last two properties?

Simple: DO NOT attempt to dry out damp coke in an oven, it will form little rubber lumps of useless crap and ruin your frying pan.

You may be less interested to hear that 'On hydrolysis with mineral acids or baryta, cocaine breaks up into ecgonine (tropine carboxylic acid), benzoic acid and methyl alcohol, being closely related to atropine.'

This information dates from the days when Chemistry GCSE used cocaine in its field experiments as often as anhydrous copper sulphate.

For obvious reasons the tradition is not carried on with the kids of today.

MORE COKE FACTS FROM THE JAZZ AGE:

It was first synthesised in 1923 by Willstatter and Bode (who it's a fair guess drove around in an open-topped Model 'T' with a bass-boosted gramaphone, dripping in Rene Lalique jewellery).

It is interesting to note that even back in the 1930s it was fair to say: 'most of the cocaine of commerce is a partially synthetic product'. So when your man mixes your £60 gram with three parts £1.99 Persil auto, don't think he's not following in a grand tradition.

Cocaine, apparently, 'produces little or no action on the unbroken skin, but if it is injected subcutaneously, or applied to mucus membranes such as those of the mouth, eye, nose, complete anaesthesia is produced.'

Thus if anyone fancies rubbing it in their eyes or injecting it under the fingernails then they have the medical go-ahead.

'A 5-10% solution is sufficient to abolish pain and touch, but stronger solutions are required to abolish sensations of heat and cold.

'If cocaine be swallowed its anaesthetic properties act on the mucous membrane of the stomach; the sensation of hunger is deadened and, therefore, persons taking the drug by the mouth can go for a long period without feeling the want of food.'

Most familiar will be the sentence: 'The central nervous system is first stimulated and later depressed.'
The tome recommends: 'Moderate doses increase

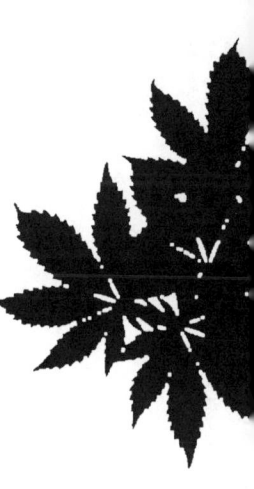

the bodily and mental power and give a sense of calmness and happiness; fatigue is abolished.

'Long exhausting feats can be carried out under the greater bodily power produced, and the inhabitants of Peru chew the coca leaves for this reason. A single large dose [= "fat line"] causes mental excitement, delirium, ataxy, with headache and depression later.'

That just about sums it up, along with the little-known fact that 'A cocaine spray is often used to spray the throats of sensitive persons before making a laryngeal examination.'

So come over all sensitive next time you visit your laryngealist for a check-up, and you might be lucky enough to feel that sweet, sweet bitterness running down your windpipe.

Remember: as the Encyclopaedia says, 'In Europe it is practically never used for its restorative effect, only for its anaesthetic properties: it is not a food, the good it does being only temporary.'

Wise words indeed.

A USER-FRIENDLY GUIDE

How to take CRACK

Once you have successfully located a source of crack, and negotiated its purchase without injury, you're already over the hard part. Thousands of addicts struggling to kick the habit might choose to disagree, but that's to worry about later. Crack is a simple drug to use, and there need be no mystery about it. A little custom-made pipe is all very well, but for an authentic scuzzy hit one must use a crumpled drinks can.

THE TWELVE STEPS

Step 1
Purchase a canned soft drink and calmly drink the contents (careful with your choice here - if this is your first time, anything unpleasant you ingest might make a surprise reappearance later, so the likes of Tizer, Vimto or Vegetable V8 are right out).

Step 2
Holding the can upright in your left hand, rotate your wrist 90 degrees so the can becomes horizontal. Make sure the pull-hole is pointing downwards, at 6 o'clock on the aluminium face.

Step 3
When you're sure everything is correctly aligned, squeeze the can gently to create a crease. You need to sculpt a concave surface such as will retain the rocks.

Step 4
Take a school compass, rusty nail or sharp knife in your right hand and proceed to perforate the topside of the can. Make four or five small holes in a cluster along the crease, not so close as to breach into each other but close enough to create an efficient 'drag'. Again, make sure the holes are no bigger than the rocks.

Step 5
Light a cigarette and breathe in the noxious fumes. Enjoy it, since this will seem like fresh air compared to the toxic gas you are preparing yourself to inhale.

Step 6
You're halfway to heaven. After a couple of drags, you will have about 1cm of ash on the end of your cancer stick. This should be the perfect amount to make a little 'nest' for your precious eggs. Crack-eggs, that is.

Step 7
Instead of tapping off the excess into an ashtray or onto your host's carpet, caress the ash into the ridge and pat down with the end of your cigarette until you have created some attractive 'bedding' material.

Step 8
Now unwrap your wee bag of joy and remove a decent-sized rock. Split if necessary using a kitchen knife, making sure not to shatter the crystal or scatter the shards.

Step 9
Pick out the choice pieces, which should be around the size of ball-bearings or small bogies

(in the US, 'boogers'). Lower them lovingly onto the ash clustered around the holes – two or three at a time will be ample.

Step 10
Holding the can in your left hand and a cigarette lighter in your right, move the aperture to your lips with a steady arm and suck manfully as you lick the flame against the rocks. Look out for the tell-tale 'sizzle' which indicates your flame has struck gold.

Step 11
Wince as a combination of crack, old ash and burnt aluminium (plus whatever the hell your man cooked it with) all congregate in your lungs. The taste should be reassuringly bitter and metallic. Pass the can to a friend as you sit down and rub your eyes.

Step 12
Repeat until you get no more change out of the blackened rocks. This may entail two or three successful 'takes', depending on the size of the rock. The great thing about crack is, when you're ready for more, just chuck another log on the fire. If you use the bag and STILL require more, simply withdraw more money and go off in search of your guy. Repeat and fade.

HANDY HINT
Get used to following a 'Twelve Step' system such as this one. You may find it useful practice for when in due course you are introduced to another, more famous one, as a direct result of your abuse of this book.

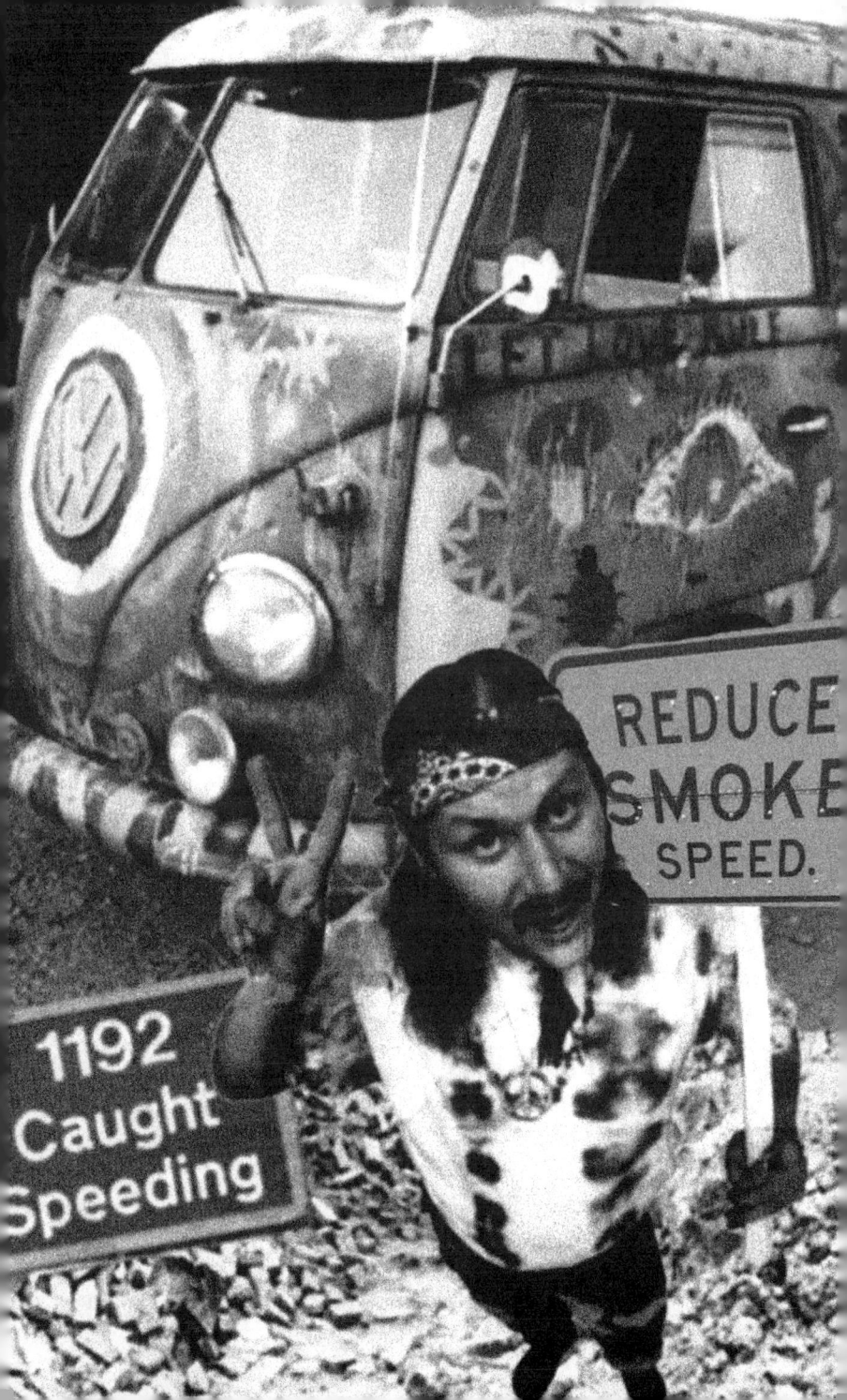

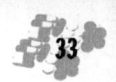

How to take SPEED

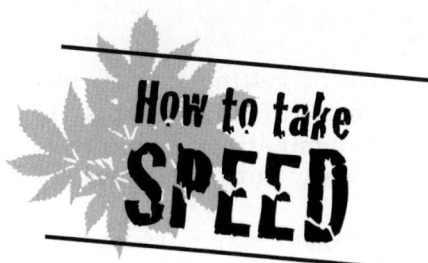

In a word: DON'T.

It's deeply unfashionable and uncool; to be classified with solvents (see later).

Like glue, it will make you spotty and retarded and its effects do not justify the undertaking.

Having said that, in its defence it is extremely cheap.

In fact it is true of most drugs that the effects never justify the concomitant side-effects (ill-health, bad skin, poverty and mental collapse).

But reminding people of this tends to take away the fun, so we'll run with speed anyway.

It also provides a welcome opportunity to describe the making of a wrap, a skill which you will need as and when you graduate to cocaine.

For this you will need something stronger than paper and thinner than card. Choose sheets from a magazine rather than a newspaper, perhaps a weekend pull-out section: the glossy surface will be less greedily absorbent of your precious purchase. Also the risk of getting newsprint on your powder is averted (though this is singularly less contaminating then most of the stuff they actually put in the powder).

Porno cards from phone boxes provide a witty medium for your fun; even better, try the omnipresent National Lottery cards. It is difficult to pinpoint at precisely what point in the last 2 years they became the single biggest carrier of speed, heroin and cocaine.

In any event, they act as an amusing reminder of what the drugs industry really is: a tax on the poor and stupid.

> First you must fashion it into a perfect square. If you are still at school, or if that is where most of your deals are made, then you will be readily equipped with a ruler or set square.
>
> Fold one corner of a larger sheet back on to itself, creating a triangle with edges of around 3-4 inches.
>
> Then tear along the side or sides of the sheet where it forms a flap, using the hard edge of your geometry equipment/ switchblade/ CD case.
>
> Unfold the triangle, and you have a perfect square, with a perfect ridge along the middle.
>
> Practice the origami aspect of the next stage BEFORE you crumble in the powder/rocks, in case you should fuck it up.
>
> Simply fold back into the triangle, then grasp the two facing 'ears' and fold them back into each

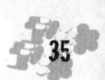

other, leaving about an inch and a half between the new creases.

If you've done the maths right (ie the two sides aren't longer than the centre, but overlap enough most of the way) then you should be able to tuck one point into the vaginal folds of the other.

This sealed, crease and fold the remaining point, leaving a perfect rectangle sealed in the centre, and tuck it into the welcoming cradle.

All told, this is much easier than tying a bow-tie.

Speed is more usually dabbed in a wetted finger than 'enjoyed' in lines.

Even better, mix it into a jelly mould for parties, and tell guests it's just 'vodka jelly'. Then watch as their eyes start to pop and they gasp for air later in the evening. It will make your guests vivacious, chatty, aggressive and uncontrollable – all the right ingredients for an inexpensive knees-up, and they will thank you for it.

The same, please note, does NOT apply for hallucinogens or rhypnol. Both may land you in serious trouble with your friends, your wife and the law.

See also: Crystal Meth, made popular in the US for frat parties and trailer parks.

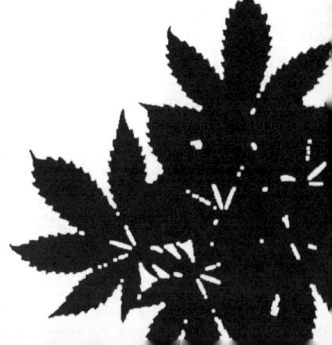

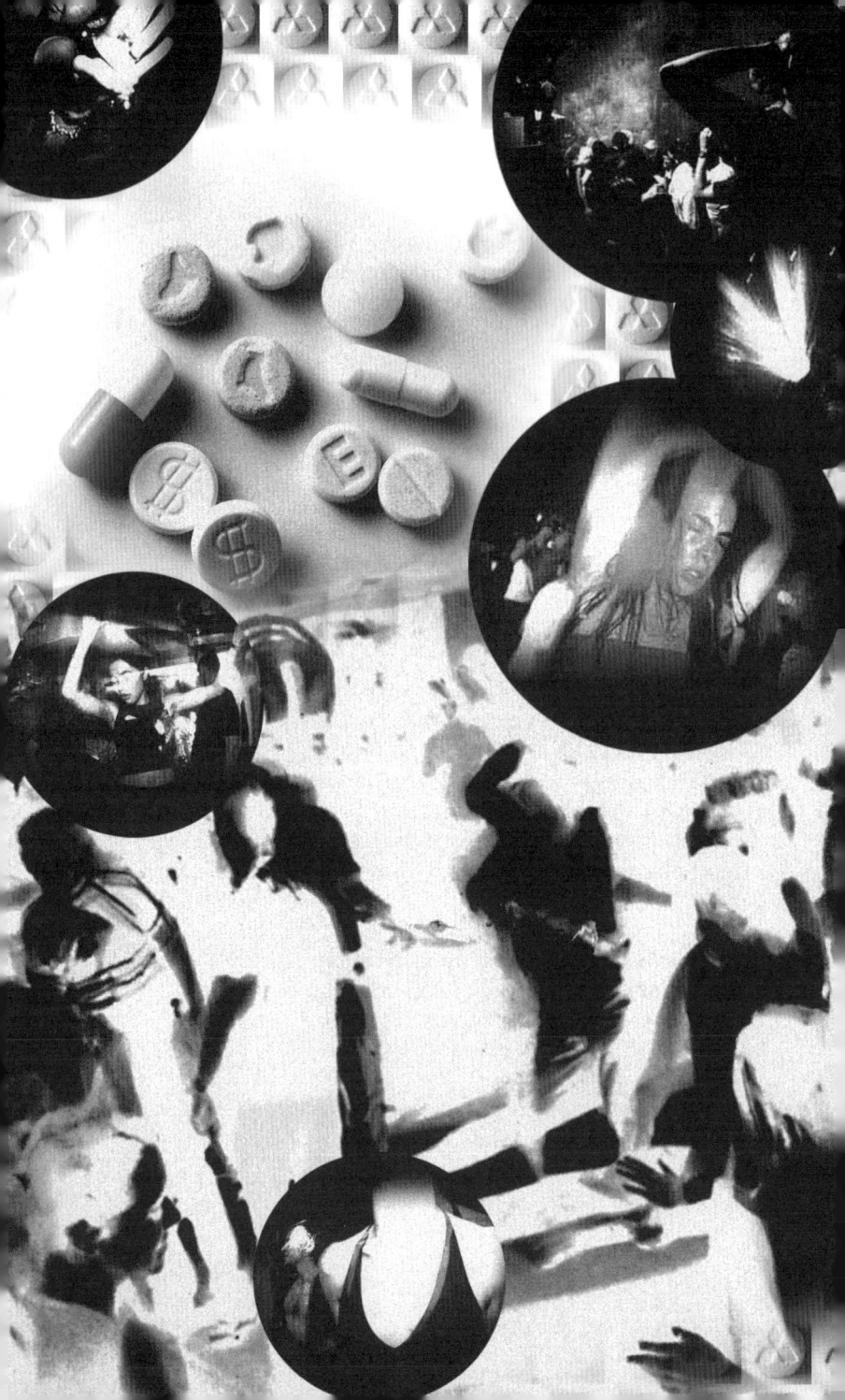

How to take ECSTASY

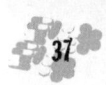

Now this is a funny one. Legend has it that this is the drug that makes you want to hug complete strangers and make love to the entire planet.

This can be true, but it is equally likely to be the drug that makes you gurn in the corner, shaking your head and talking to a teapot.

The good (intended effect) stuff in an 'E' is Methylenedioxymethylamphetamine, a word with which to impress friends that also scores a massive 70 in Scrabble.

(Plus chances are you'd use up all your letters, so that's an extra 50 points straight away. Sadly its more common label, MDMA, is not acceptable as it is an abbreviation.)

'Coming up' is characterised by a popping of the ears and sudden feeling of weightlessness.

Other people's conversations, even your own voice, will all become echo-y and gradually merge into some kind of background soundtrack – unless of course you're in a loud club, as most people are, in which case you won't notice the difference.

The music will appear to loop on the same two bars for the rest of the evening, but you won't mind: in fact you'll think it's the best thing you've ever heard.

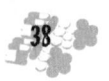

This is how shit-for-brains club DJs manage to make a living.

The emotional effects are more complicated.

HOW TO TAKE ECSTASY

The evening spent on ecstasy begins with a sweaty handshake, a surreptitious transfer of palm to mouth... and a horribly bitter taste.

Doctors will assure you that the pissy ammonia fizzing on your taste-buds is 'just the active ingredient, mate', but since the actual MDMA is diluted by about 200,000,000 parts chalk, it does seem like a horrible joke at your expense.

I suspect ecstasy is flavoured deliberately by the lab jokers back in Holland out of sheer jealousy because they don't get out that much.

Of course, if you have a drink handy, you can get the little bastards down with minimum contact to the absorbent parts of your mouth; but it's harder when you're enjoying a crumbly half with a friend, especially if you lose the toss and have to bite it in two.

Ecstasy does like to encourage that kind of caring, sharing mentality – plus halving an E in today's marketplace works out cheaper than letting someone scab a fag.

An even more disgusting method is to

How to do Drugs

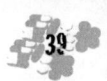

'crunch up' a pill on your molars. The received wisdom on this is, 'quicker rush mate'.

It's true, it will provoke an almost instant reaction – most likely an attack of the shivers. You'll end up with lots of little grains of bitterness lodged in your back teeth, which you'll be discovering with your tongue for long afterwards, and this is the quickest way to induce gakking.

There is, of course, a yet more disgusting way to take ecstasy.

THE BUM RUSH or,
'You can stick your suppositories up your arse'.

The notorious 'bum rush' gets a bum rap from me. Not that it isn't worth trying. The sad fact is, there comes a time in every mash-head's career that the drugs just aren't as quick anymore.

You can take two, four, ten pills in a night... but somehow the effect is never as big as your first half all those years ago. The veterans mutter that the pills were better back in the Hacienda '89.

The younger bores talk in hushed tones about when 'Bishis'* first turned up to revitalise the scene.

But one way or another, everyone agrees the kick is getting smaller.

*BISHIS mitsubishis, so called because of the corporate logo reappropriated by the manufacturers to decorate the revolutionary, stronger pill that emerged in the late '90s and 'saved clubland', according to the same people who claim they only really care about the music.

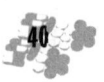

So what are you gonna do? Well, whatever anyone sensible would do: stick it up your arse, of course.

'It's like your first time,' the seedy-looking man grins at your shoulder.

If he means it's like the first time you've had something uncomfortable shoved up your rectum, he's right.

Once there, the pill should be absorbed directly into the bloodstream via the soft intestinal wall.

Or alternately, it'll sit there just inside the colon sulking for hours, and after some irritable attempts to sit down you'll have to fish it out, wash it clean and pop it down the usual way.

Don't gag, it's your own arse after all.

Many pills bear a distinctive 'branding' logo: the letter E, the apple, the 'happy eater'. The irony of parodying corporate identity is that the products also rely on branding for exactly the same reason – market forces.

Brand confidence affects the black market too. When a batch of 'green apples' was associated with a high-profile death and tabloid campaign, they slipped off the streets; when word of mouth got round about the 'bishi, it was all anyone ever asked for. Like 'biro' or 'hoover', it became a brand that stood for a whole concept.

How to do Drugs

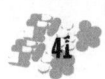

> Rumour had it that the UK Marketing Director of Mitsubishi made no effort to discourage the trade, as it meant widespread brand visibility and association with a high-quality product. Some people will even tell you the Japanese company was actually behind the scheme. But then, people on drugs will believe anything.

FIELD NOTES

An inevitable ceremony on any E-vening is the 'duds' routine. Here's how it works:

7.00pm
Your mate's weird friend opens the bag and passes them round.

7.05pm
You wait until everyone's got one and then drop them together.

7.15pm
You secretly make it a double-drop just in case.

8.00pm
A few tinnies to the good, the gang decide to hit Yates's Wine Lodge. Things are only a little fuzzy.

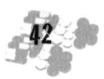

8.20pm
A growing suspicion: that no-good dealer's fucking skanked you.

8.30pm
A voice in your ear. 'These are duds mate.' You shake your head vigorously in agreement. 'Shall we take the rest of them?'

8.34pm
Oh fuck, they're NOT duds

8.36pm
This is brilliant. This is really happening.

8.39pm
Oh shit... I didn't really just drop another five did I?

5.23am
Come round in someone's kitchen

Chemical logic is on display at its finest here. If the pills really were bogus, would it even have made sense to do another one? Or another seven?

The fact is, something within you knows, the drugs are gonna work. It's not there yet but it's in the post. You're just frustrated and you want it now.

Well, like your nanny told you what you want you don't always get. E can take anything from half an hour to an hour and a half before it kicks in. But there's no better way to ensure you come up on an E than by taking another one.

Part of this, of course, is Sod's Law. But science may play its part too. Perhaps your senses are shaken out of neutral by the shock of that vile taste on your tongue again.

Most likely, though, it's the giddy rush of chemical enthusiasm – consistent with being just about to come up – that makes you think it would be such a great idea to pop another.

A note on Gurning

This phenomenon is also associated with cocaine, but it's E that makes it an art form.

You may well wake up the next morning with chewed-up cheeks and a swollen tongue, spitting blood and feathers, alone.

If so, then you can be sure the reason you didn't pull was that you spent half the night pulling faces, wincing and chomping on your jaw.

This is particularly painful if you grind your teeth habitually at night, your teeth jut out unevenly, or you have your wisdom teeth coming through at awkward angles.

Fortunately, enamel is only so strong, so in time you'll grind the little fellas down into line. Who needs them anyway?

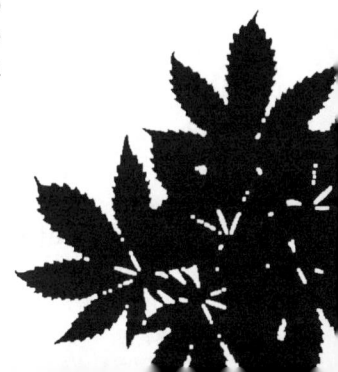

Variations on a theme

MDMA Powder

I'm sure there are purists who think this stuff is cheating, and that somehow, by making E like cocaine you're betraying the spirit of the second summer of love. Yes – but it's also guaranteed free of those awkward two-day comedowns.

That, coupled with the fact it comes in those much-loved wraps, makes it ideal fodder for the work-hard-play-hard city trader. Consequently, the dealer can charge what the hell he likes. Everybody's happy.

2CI's (ALSO CALLED 2CB's, ICI's, JCB's, GOD KNOWS WHAT ELSE)

Ah, the '**Willy Wonka**' drug. These babies are what people call 'very trippy', and come in all shapes and colours, sometimes with blue speckles – you know, like those mints you can't buy anymore because the government said they looked like drugs.

I liken them to the work of Willy Wonka not because of any unfortunate side-effects in the bedroom (SEE SEX AND DRUGS) but because of the magical journey they take you on.

Remember the gum that turned Violet Beauregard into a blueberry? You popped it into your mouth, then went through a pleasant sequence of starter, main course and finally a surprisingly twisted dessert.

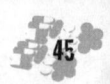

Well, that's pretty much the experience of taking these acid-laced pills.

The first course is merely an amuse-bouche, just the happy sensation that they start taking effect a bit quicker than regular pills: a little bit like having taken a line of powder, very gentle, very pleasant.

Then you come up - and you come up big. This is the meat-and-two-veg of the operation, the thing you really bought the pill for, and it will leave most gourmands wholly satisfied.

Sadly you probably won't have left room for pudding. This is the time when you really do start turning into a blueberry.

The first time I took one of these I'd been happily dining for hours on the MDMA course before someone suggested I took a bit of a drag of their joint to help ease me down.

What followed on inhalation was to see my right hand turn black and all five fingers simply melt before drifting off into an acrid smoke.

It took hours before the Oompa-Loompas were able to drag me down from the ceiling with their horrible rakes.

HIGHLY RECOMMENDED.

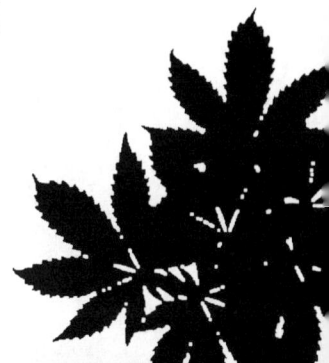

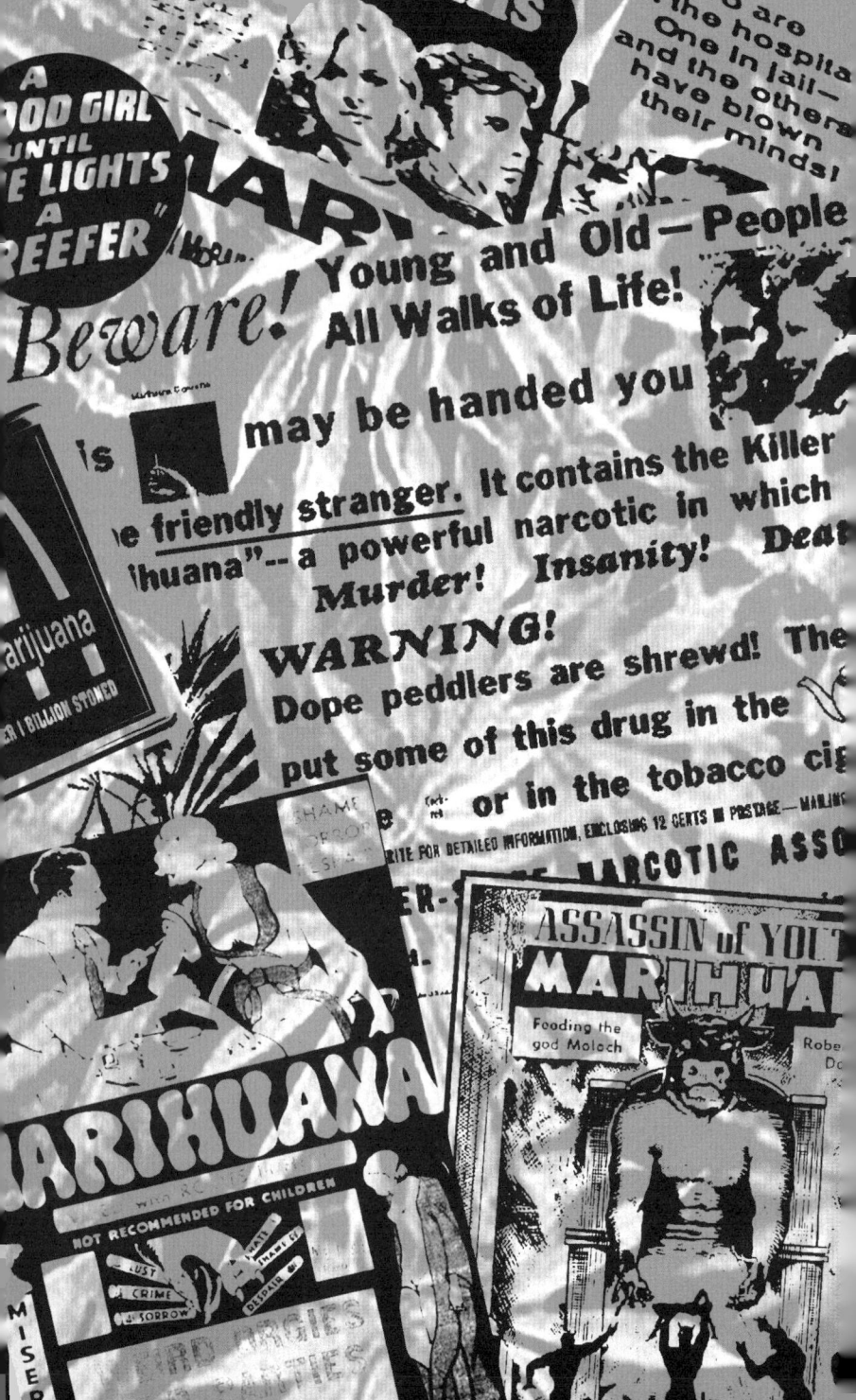

How to do MARIJUANA

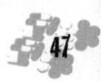

A nice easy starter pack, this, and an ideal drug to wean in children, younger brothers or ageing 'squares'.

It boasts some of the thrill of mild psychotropic properties coupled with some of the thrill of mild illegality (see 'The Law').

Think of it as a 'funsize' high, although certain forms of skunk can indeed drive you permanently insane. The closest thing to a marijuana 'overdose' will see you giggle till you're sick, perhaps falling unconscious with the permanent loss of all but a few braincells. As I said, a mild reaction.

To achieve this, please study the following diagram carefully:

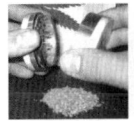 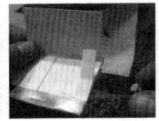 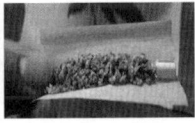 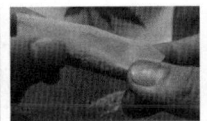 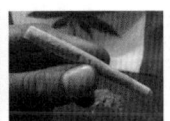

There, a handful of easy steps to rolling your first marijuana cigarette, or 'joint', and thus impressing your friends.

Be careful how many people you do this in front of, however. The trailblazer in any group

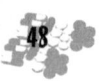

of young delinquents who first manages a joint will probably be expected to do the rolling duties for the rest of his drug-abusing career, to the extent that his or her peers will never bother to learn.

Remember, it might be cool to be the one in the corner rolling joints at parties when you're fourteen, but by your mid-twenties most people will look at you like the loser who hasn't changed his life or his haircut.

This is especially true of impressing girls, who by the time they leave university will be into more grown-up ideas of what makes a guy 'cool' – things like money, a car and a job.

The best compromise is to teach yourself secretly, so you're never stuck when on your own, but equally never viewed as designated 'dope guy'.

That poor fool must endure a social burden as great as the designated driver, and he is also usually expected to bring and share his own gear and not charge his friends per puff.

The other advantage of learning on your own is that your first efforts are not carried out – and therefore cruelly mocked – in public.

You will probably have to roll your first social joint while drunk or already stoned, so get those shaky fingers in practice.

If this is still too hard, try these handy short-cuts:

How to do Drugs

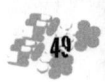

Shortcut (I)
The cheeky 'one-y'

No harder than making a rolled-up cigarette with a sprinkling of buds or crumble of resin in the mix (the only skill is to avoid burning your thumbs when cooking up the edge of the block with your flinty lighter).

If you can't even do this, then don't ever worry about trying to make a Camberwell Carrot. Equally if you CAN do this, then the same skills apply to making a proper joint, so adapt the principle to bigger fish and stop making excuses. Easy.

Shortcut (II)
The parrot's nest.

So named (by Professor Crackhead) after the Amazonian parrot's lazy shortcut to making a 'nest' by using the hollowed-out shell of an old tree-trunk.

This parrot finds a thin, hollow trunk with an open top, fills it with leaves and simply lowers itself down to lay its eggs in a ready-made tubular bed. We can learn much from Mother Nature.

What you must do is find a spare cigarette, and using a matchstick (not the poisonous end) hollow out the debris from the core, as a parrot might use its claw. Make sure not to scratch or break the paper cylinder. Then simply sprinkle in the magic dust, along with most of the tobacco mix you removed, patting it back down nice and tight as you go using the same matchstick. Hey presto – an easy and palatable joint, one you can 'prepare earlier', one even acceptable to produce from a regular packet and light up after a formal meal (providing your hosts have no sense of smell or grip on reality). Remember to store it your frugal pack of ten the wrong way up so you don't lose track, or you might just let a stranger get lucky and 'borrow' it by mistake.

Shortcut (III)
How to cheat with style.

It is possible to acquire, from certain specialist shops or less enlightened regions of the world, liquid cannabis resin in an inkpot. The cap doubles as a brush and dipping stick, rather like the equally rush-giving Tippex, so all you need do is daub the sides of a Silk Cut with a delicate glaze and allow to dry.

Fancy a fiercer smoke?
Paint it on thick with a Rothmans, allowing each layer to harden before recoating. Mmm, disgusting.

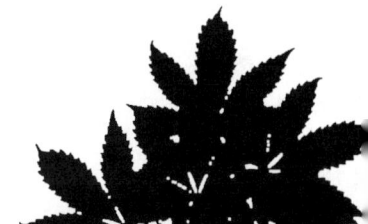

The other way to smoke is by bong or water-pipe. You can, if you prefer, use one of those fancy ethnic accessories bought on gap-years in Morocco and stag-nights in Amsterdam. They can look like ugly ceramic jugs with jutting chambers, or little leathery scrotums on the end of a length of thin hosepipe. They may well have that mass-produced handcraft finish or be decorated with a Jamaican flag and a patronising comedy rasta.

Perhaps there will be an amateurishly recreated Mona Lisa enjoying a crafty 'draw' on one side. When you have stopped laughing, sprinkle the gear on top of the chimney, using a bit of tobacco as bedding; then wrap your lips around the mouthpiece, using one hand to hold the offending object in place and the other to hold the lighter.

Use the fingers of your third hand, if you have one, to cover any 'bong-holes' that might be letting out the smoke and stopping the vacuum.

You spark the lighter on its side against the rocks of gear, and when one of them 'takes' you suck hard and long, taking two or three gulps while occasionally raising and then quickly replacing your finger on the bong-hole during breaths, rather like you're playing the recorder.

This makes you look like you know what you're doing, even though in practice it loses a bit of smoke.

You keep the stuff in your mouth for as long as you can, thereby turning your whole throat into a 'second chamber', much like the House of Lords, before inhaling.

Don't turn green and you may realise it's actually more fun than it looked. If you are using a large Turkish water-pipe you'll have felt the added kick of some nice bubbles while examining the exquisite colouring and fine craftsmanship of the object. Because of the legitimate civilian uses of such devices to smoke pleasantly-flavoured fruit tobacco, these are also acceptable in polite middle-class society as pieces of decorative furniture (except in America, the Republic of Ireland and Bhutan, where even smoking in public can have you slapped with a lawsuit).

For those who prefer a scuzzier hit, a formal, expensively-imported bong is an extravagance you can do without. Blue Peter-style, all you need is a biro, a bottle of Evian (any size) and a Kit-Kat wrapper, all available from any 24-hour garage. Chances are, if it's half midnight and that's all you're buying, you'll get a dirty look; but you can live with this.

HOW TO...
MAKE YOUR OWN BONG

Poke through the bottle with the biro about two-thirds up, without making the hole wider than the pen itself, and again on the opposite side near the top if you favour the 'blow-hole' effect.

Fill the bottle half full of water to test whether you misread the above instruction (this is where you'll realise if you've placed the holes brainlessly low). **Empty the biro of its cartridge and nib,** but don't throw away in case you have no other means of perforating the foil, or fancy doing the crossword afterwards.

Insert the pen shaft into the first hole, pointing between 30-45 degrees downwards, held in by the tension of the hole being a little tight, with the tapering end as your mouthpiece.

Remove the bottle cap, invert and place on the table in case any of your guests require a makeshift ashtray.

Then wrap the top with the silver inner packaging of your Kit-Kat, having removed the twin biscuit treat and put it aside in a cool and hygenic place for when you get suddenly hungry an hour or two later (there's no place for waste when you're making a bong on a tight budget).

Pierce the foil seal three or four time in a cluster, without weakening the structure or making a hole so big you can't rest your rocks on it.

Hey presto, return to the top of the section marked 'Bongs' and follow the simple instructions to nirvana.

The scuzziest hit of all is obtainable through tin cans (see 'crack').

How much to take..
Marijuana won't kill you through overdose.

But it might just drive you mad.

Worse still, it can kill your personality.

If you only find your friends funny on dope, try looking for new ones when you're straight enough to make a sound judgement.

Write down your conversations when fucked to peruse in the morning.

Are they still interesting? Clever? Inspired, funny or profound?

What have you actually solved in the universe? If the results aren't what you'd hoped, then adjust your dose up or down until you're worth knowing.

Avoid people who don't smoke fags but still do pot. They are self-righteous and boring. They say things like 'I save my lungs for the best' and 'grass is natural – that shit will kill you'.

They are arseholes, be they hypocrites who happily enjoy a dose of tobacco as part of their jazzier cigarette, or hardcore ganga-tarians who only smoke it in kingies, blunts or bongs.

Regular fag-smoking remains an important accompaniment to meat, fish, beer, wine and cocaine.

A dope-only dullard will probably forgo all these essential protein groups.

When chunks of grimy soap-bar resin get dull, you will duly move on to skunk and superskunk.

Then ultraskunk and googleskunk. They will have exotic names like White Widow and Golden Dragon, and they will make you spin out.

Then you will be drawn once again back to regular soap-bar as you graduate from youthful thrillseeker to slightly edgy adult who has vaguely medicinal needs for a bedtime quietener.

Suddenly you will realise that you are taking drugs not to change your state of mind but to maintain an uneasy status quo.

This is when your life is
effectively over.

Hallucinogenics

Don't be fooled by the name: hallucinogenic drugs do not necessarily make you HALLUCINATE.

At least, not in the way it might be depicted in a cartoon or a Shakespearean love-comedy. 'Hallucinations' do not usually entail giant pink giraffes and fluffy castles in the sky. More likely, you'll be staring for hours at the patterns in the linoleum flooring of someone's kitchen, or gawping at the wallpaper in the loo, waiting for it to drip.

Equally you might 'hallucinate' that someone doesn't like you, or does, or is ignoring you, or staring at you, or OH GOD WHEN WILL IT STOP?

You see, if you're expecting fireworks, visions and waking dreams, you might be disappointed. Stories of people jumping out of windows believing they could fly are (usually) exaggerated, perhaps by the nanny state/ arrogant liberal media/ right-wing do-gooders in Whitehall who want to frighten their subjects from taking any drugs other than those that the Treasury gets a cut.

Some people do experience this kind of thing, others find their brains fight too hard for control to really let go. But don't feel too disappointed to be in the second category: you'll be grateful when you make it through the night without going insane.

Also, not all drugs that make you hallucinate are classed as hallucinogenics. THC, the active ingredient in dope, will do the job: super-skunk is as likely to set you off as anything. Then there's MDMA, which often hits the mark: if you combine it with strong sleeping pills, jellies especially, that's the best formula for waking dream-like states. In fact most of the time you actually WILL be passing in and out of sleep, so make sure you've also taken enough cocaine to keep you half-awake for the show.

So, let's look at the culprits. They basically come down to magic mushrooms and acid.

MAGIC MUSHROOMS

These fungi may not change your world-view forever, but you can certainly be assured of laughing more than you can ever remember.

LEGALITY

Perhaps the funniest thing about mushrooms is that they're legal. Or rather, they're not. Hang on, are they? The truth is that the early 21st Century saw a new summer of love, when thousands of law-abiding citizens would

How to do Drugs

spend warm days in the park spinning out on powerful hallucinogens while rozzers happily looked on with approval. How we laughed at their tit hats and petty corruption, how they loved to indulge these young hippies and their wacky ways, eager even to join in except that they were 'on duty, sir'.

Well, that all changed at the end of summer 2005. Hearing word that certain young people were 'having fun', successive Home Secretaries Blunkett and Clarke realised something would have to be done and sealed up the loophole. Portobello market no longer gaily advertises 'Magic Mushies' at a penny a bag from any of its stalls. File them alongside firecrackers and throwing stars and other harmless toys that schoolkids now have to go to mainland Europe to get their hands on.

The good news is, you can still harvest them legally from a field near you (that's assuming you live near a field). Drive out to the country in, ooh, September or so - sometime when it's warm but damp. Find a meadow full of cowpats and sneak through at night with a torch, looking for caps with all the zeal of a German commandant hunting escaped POWs by searchlight. Even better, get up very early when it's still light – an added advantage is, you can see the cows (although the farmer might be able to see you).

Concerned you might pick up the wrong cap and end up poisoning yourself? Here is a failsafe guide to what you are looking for:

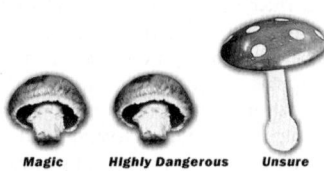

Magic   Highly Dangerous   Unsure

RECIPES

The only technical distinction between what makes a 'shroom legal or villainous is its preparation: i.e., fresh produce is a natural resource provided by Mother Earth for us all to enjoy, but anything cooked, dried or extracted is an 'evil trade in death' (argument copyright the **Daily Mail**). With this in mind, here are a number of ways to prepare mushrooms – thus putting your mind at rest if you worried for a minute you might be wasting your time on something legal.

Mushroom tea (disgusting)

Pizza al funghi (vile)

Mushroom omelette (horrid)

Mushroom jelly (awful)

Mushrooms 'au naturel' (inedible)

That's right, all these attempts to make the disgusting things more palatable are basically a waste of time (and mushrooms) – especially since the cooking process tends to take out the active ingredients.

That's why stewing or brewing is the only feasible culinary route, but unfortunately you have to be prepared to drink the horrible juice. Don't believe anyone who says they're 'just another ingredient' to be used in cooking like any other delicious mushroom; this person I guarantee will be a TERRIBLE cook.

EFFECTS

You'll see, you simple fool. You'll see.

If you manage to avoid gagging while cramming the chewy things into your dry, dry throat – and as a result don't feel sick throughout the entire trip – good luck and happy giggles. Try to avoid making the obvious 'mushroom' puns – they're not 'funghi' and are likely to bring the group down. Don't panic if you don't know any jokes – almost everything else will be funny, so that's OK.

If you're on pre-packaged stuff, supposedly there are big differences from brand to brand. 'Philosophers Stones' (a borderline immoral attempt to crack on to the under-9 Harry Potter market) are tiny and crunchy like those green fizzy sweets, and supposedly offer you 'powerful and deep insights' (i.e. laughing at things on the telly). 'Salvia Divinorum' (or, 'spit of God') hail from Mexico and offer peyote voodoo insights into the spirit land of your forefathers (i.e., laughing at more things on the telly).

The fact is yes, some are trippier and some are gigglier, but this all varies with dose and you're just as likely to spin out by overdosing on one as the other.

The only way you're gonna find out what you like is by trying them all: just be careful to count the stems and don't do the whole bag before you've had a couple of hours to see how the first lot are working. Then you can make a mature decision about whether it's what you really want with your evening. And then eat the whole bag.

ACID

Longer, stronger and generally less funny than mushrooms. Which is not to say that you won't laugh like a mad angry Jack Nicholson for the first, ooh, 3 hours. It's just that, well, you don't want to be there when the laughter stops.

Acid can sometimes bring out the nastier sides to people's characters: the side that likes to mess with other people's brains, the side that likes to spike the unwary, the side that looks like a scaly reptile with devils' eyes. It's also like a long-term commitment where the mushroom is a one-night stand; be prepared to lose 8 to 12 hours to the dark side.

Be prepared to swallow and forget everything you know. Don't even think about having anything to do the next day, like move your car or start a new job. And don't fool yourself that you actually really know anyone you're out with, because you'll never see them in quite the same way again.

Still, there are advantages. I think. It's cheap, surprisingly so given the many hours of good value misery it's going to cause. At three pounds a throw for the privilege of losing half a day to madness, that's, what, only 25p per hour of being fucked and incapable.

And it's largely undetectable by sniffer dogs and teachers. It's available in blotting tabs, droplets like peppercorns and liquid form (the latter is the easiest to misjudge – make sure you have a reliable pipette for single-drop doses).

And don't be fooled by the classic acid paranoia – that everybody else must be aware of how high you are because you've so obviously gone crazy.

Remember that they're not seeing the world as weirdly as you are. And your brain is working overtime to try and make sense of it all.

Just be confident and try to finish sentences. Apologise if you lose your thread or frighten your dinner companion, but at no point slip under and admit you may have taken acid. It may sound like a reasonable excuse to you, but to a straight this will make you seem a lot more dangerous and threatening than just the harmless eccentric they had taken you for.

If all this sounds too much like hard work, well, yes it is. It may seem hilarious to take acid in social situations but then it will rapidly start to feel like the longest day of your life. You start to see the world from so many angles that it becomes hard to describe them all; you can see where your conversation's heading so far ahead that you'll lose track of where you are. It's much better to take when you don't need to pretend to hold it together. On a beach, in a park, on a parachute jump... that kind of thing.

DMT

A strange one, this. On paper it's a very strong, very lucid trip that only lasts about 15 minutes.

What could be better? On the minus side, a worrying number of daytrippers experience identical nightmares, namely the sudden realisation that little green men have been living among us for many years – and one only has to pop DMT to start seeing them.

For this reason it became the official drug of the Raelians, a David-Icke-style conspiracy religion predicated on a belief that we are merely a slave race to an ancient group of lizard-like extraterrestrials. And for THAT reason, we cannot in good conscience recommend the drug in this book.

Paraphernalia

We've already covered the 'bong' and the 'crack pipe'. Here's some other 'totally rad' stuff you might need:

THE BULLET
(for use with powdered drugs)

Ideal for circumventing the whole malarkey with lines and credit cards and pub toilets, also for clubs with no surfaces in the loos or simply greedy toilet attendants who want to spray your hands with perfume but to whom you don't want to be shamed into giving money. Here's how it works.

Basically just hold between thumb and forefinger and twist your hands like you know what you're doing. As long as one hand's holding the knob and you cover the blow-hole with your finger it usually seems to work. You can check whether it's ready by the tasty little preview that will have gathered on your fingertip.

These are highly convenient for discreet sniffing in social situations, e.g. at the table, in the Royal Box at Wimbledon and so on. They come in one and two gram sizes. A full top chamber will provide one hit.

THE WATERPROOF WRAP

A new innovation from Manhattan. Much better to drop drunkenly down the u-bend than your average lottery ticket wrap, and less likely on hot days to let the stuff go soggy in your pocket. Essential next year in Ibiza, a bit of a luxury in London.

THE POPPER

A medium for amyl nitrate, these are just little bottles of evil-smelling liquid. It is a powerful 'relaxant' and a bringer of headaches, so is thus equally practical as an anal sex aid for the willing OR a tailor-made excuse if you decide you'd really rather not. Remove the cap and hold to one nostril. Then try the other. Remember to reseal the crap bottle top before you black out and drop the thing, it evaporates easily. Do not try to drink.

SILVER/GOLD STRAWS/BOXES

You know the sort of thing – like cigarette cases, only with chambers for storing joints or coke. The height of pretension.

SICK BUCKET

A classic design, still useful for first-time heroin users.

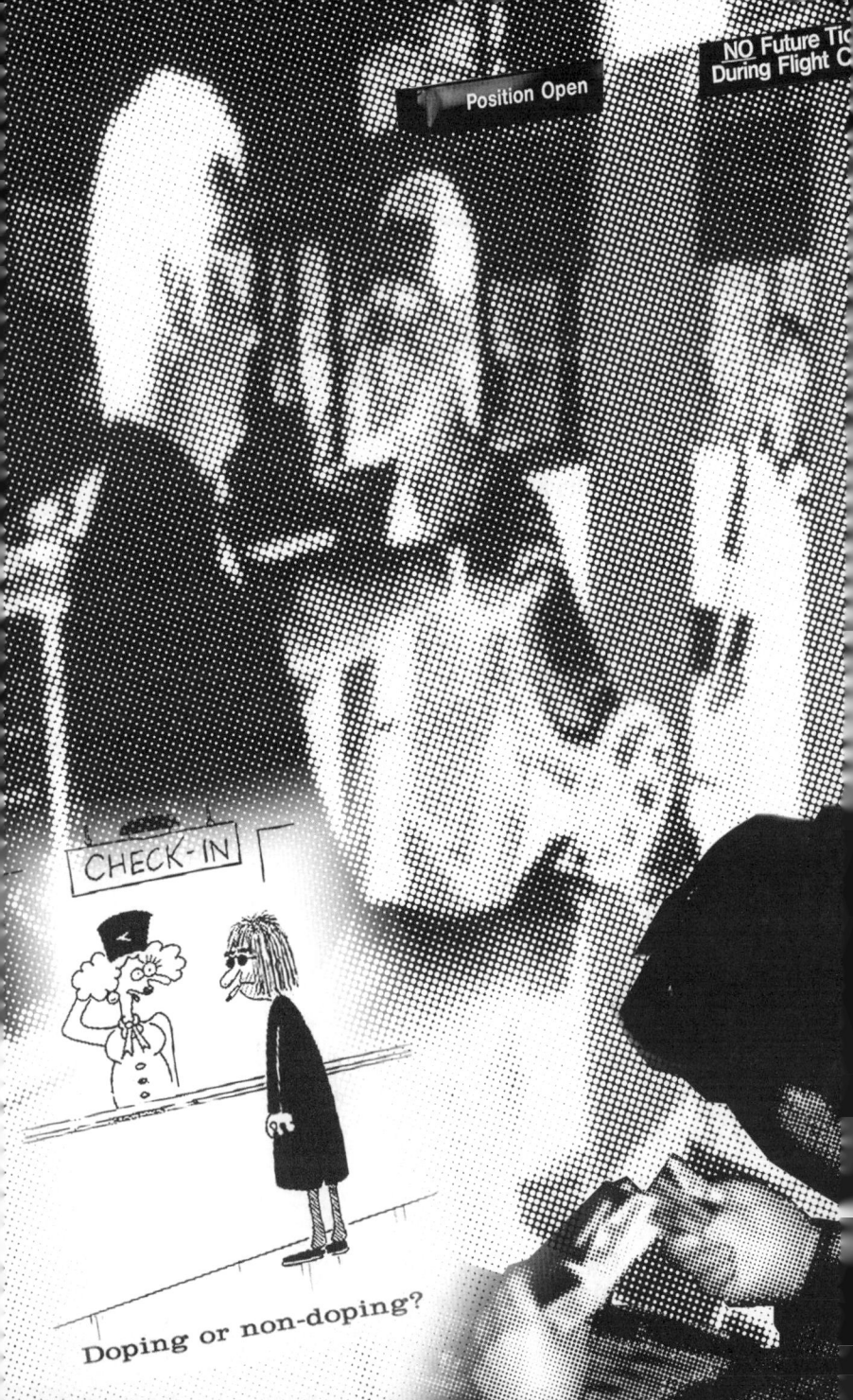

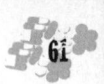

Smuggling

Howard Marks has earned a whole cult for himself by breaking international trade laws.

Personally, I couldn't give a fuck about the guy, but then you're only entitled to the heroes you deserve.

Smuggling is generally carried out either by ruthless criminals, or idiots like you and me; in the latter case, most often accidentally.

I'm not just talking about being thrown into a Third World jail for carrying home your new boyfriend's ethnic fertility keepsake in your hand luggage.

There's also the huge number of people who wander through customs with half a wrap still in their wallet, or a couple of pills and maybe a lump of hash rolling around their pockets.

And miraculously, they get away with it – probably because they're still in a highly 'relaxed' state and are giving off the amiable vibes of someone beyond suspicion.

This is the paradox of successful smuggling, whereby only someone stupid enough not to be worried can usually pull it off.

Try to project the confidence of the calmest people on the plane: the air stewards, who of course never let their

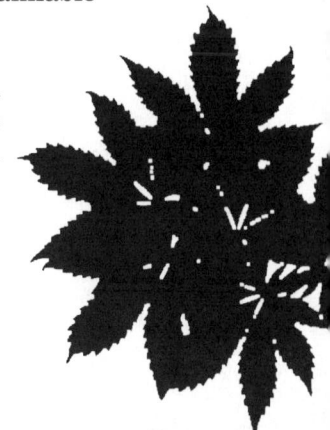

hair down at destinations like Rio or Ibiza, and never take advantage of express check-in to carry their party home with them. Or swagger through like the ever-sober pilots, who just like any other passenger would certainly not be allowed onto a flight whilst obviously under the influence.

These are the blameless sorts of people who'll never get their turbans turned out at check-in.

To help foster self-confidence, be creative. Consider bold plans for concealing magic mushrooms within regular cooking ingredients, like sandwich filling or pizza topping. Or try a false bottom (no, to your suitcase, not your arse, on which more later).

> Along with personal flair, a bit of subtlety is called for. Bathroom products, say tubes of hairgel or jars of wax, are good hiding places for moderate weights of gear – **but make it too subtle, like in a pot of talcum powder, and you may have lost your stash for good.**

As with actually taking drugs, if you're feeling really adventurous you can use your cavities.

Swallowing a condom full of the

merchandise is the stuff of urban legend – as is the consequence of the sheath splitting once inside you (ask your local Catholic priest and he'll tell you that always happens, boom-boom).

Chances are the johnny will come through your system without provoking a mid-air heart attack, providing you remembered to tie the end up, but if you do make it you've still got to fish about in the toilet the other end.

Another method is to sit on the stuff, aided by your favourite cavity (men only really have one choice here).

My mother always taught me the following rhyme:

> **'If you're dealing with wraps,**
> **stick it in your flaps.**
> **If it's pills or glue, your arse will do.'**

Tragically my stepsister suffered a terrible accident following the latter advice on glue too closely – doctors quite literally had to tear her a new arsehole.

It seems one of the three substances was only included in the mnemonic for the purposes of a rhyme... but the adage still holds fast when it comes to the other methods. Clearly girls have an easier time of it accommodating wide, flat wraps, providing they meet with polite body searches.

As for pills, you can't just stuff a whole bag up there, so some cunning is called for.

Here are some Ikea-style instructions for the 'Swizzlers' technique, based on the popular children's sweet. Amyl Nitrate may help you relax into this one:

1. Stack the pills nose-to-tail, like any regular fizzy sweet packet, and wrap in clingfilm.

2. Bunch the ends up like a christmas cracker, and seal tight at the neck using a standard lighter.

3. Once the plastic is melted airtight and left to cool, ease slowly up the hole. Re-apply pants.

Watch out for chafing from those crumpled ends! You might want to make sure it's a smoother ride by folding one end over and sellotaping flat: that is, the business end.

It is advisable to keep at least the tail of the other end poking out, for ease of removal – take a tip from tampon manufacturers here.

When airborne, once the passenger seatbelt light is extinguished you may wish to give your butt a rest by extracting the object for an hour or two. Or you may be enjoying it (depending on your idea of a holiday).

The truth is, even post-9/11 you can probably stroll through most airports with drugs in your sock and you won't be stopped, ooh, 9 out of 11 times.

If you like those odds, go ahead with it. The risks of getting caught tend to increase in line with the brutality of the local custodial conditions – I'm told that Thai police dogs can sniff out a Viagra in a pot of ketchup.

And the clever mutts' reward for this loyal service in this part of the world? Most likely they'll end up in a casserole.

It makes you sick.

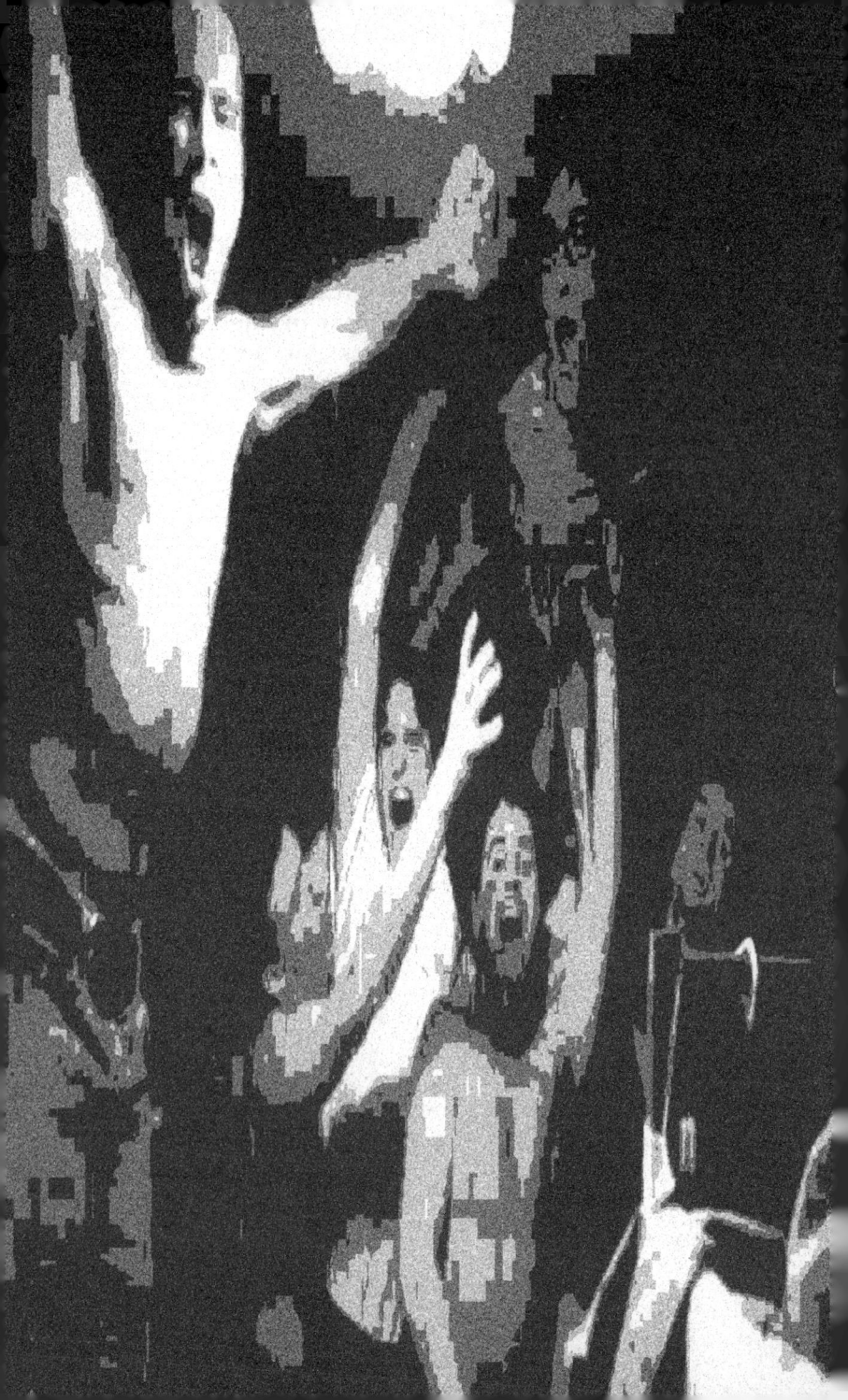

SOCIAL SCORING

The quickest and easiest way to score is through a friend.

Where to find drugs & HOW TO SCORE

If not a proper friend who deals drugs, this can just as easily be a drug dealer respectable enough to pass off among your friends.

Someone who's always bound to be carrying, and mysteriously gets invited to all the parties (except, of course, Weddings and Christenings).

While not the moral or legal loophole some would like to think it is, this sort of 'doing a mate a favour' arrangement does remove a lot of the rough edges from a drug deal.

These include:

(i) going somewhere inconvenient or unpleasant,

(ii) talking to someone frightening,

(iii) handling large quantities of money, and

(iv) feeling responsibility for checking quality, price and volume whilst smiling weakly at a man whose integrity you would not wish to question without a SAS bodyguard.

Some people, however, like these rough edges. Indeed, many would consider it important to share in this experience at least once – like visiting a city farm to show your children where milk and eggs come from.

Once you've got your hands dirty, you may even find you have a taste for it: the position of power over your friends... the rush of returning to the warm, safe party with little bags of happiness... the attention you then receive all night from men and women alike... perhaps even the small profit you think it's OK to skim off the top, to cover your expenses and risk...

This is when you are becoming a drug dealer.

Tread carefully.

Remember that after a while your friends will start inviting you to the after-party and not the main event, the dancing but not the dinner.

When you start receiving invitations asking you not to bother arriving before midnight, or your host arranges to meet after work in a Tube Station, that's when you know you've stepped over the line from friend to drug mule.

The best solution is not to rely on other people for drugs OR have people habitually relying on you. Be self-sufficient but not notorious.

Make contacts by being there or thereabouts when the deal goes down – but remember always to stay in the mindset of a punter. Whenever you are present at a drug deal, ask for an introduction.

You may get a number, you may just familiarise the pusher with your name or your voice.

Hang off respectfully and slightly awkwardly, making noises like 'Safe' and 'Sound' and 'Nice One' and 'Cool' until you are no longer perceived as a threat so much as another potential mug.

Remember it is no bad thing to be a mug.

Everyone who pays dealer prices for drugs is a mug. The prices are inflated by the stealth taxes of extortion, risk and greed.

They are almost never value-for-money in terms of the high they give you versus the trouble they cause. This is not the point.

People like drugs, they're fun, and they're willing to pay for them, especially when drunk and happy (even more so when sober and desperately unhappy – see Addiction).

All drug dealers like to feel the client can offer them something: everyone in their phone book is a soft touch, and you're not going to be attractive to pushers if you don't want to admit it.

Still, this doesn't mean you should establish yourself as the mug of mugs. Make sure your first transaction with a new man is at the right price and of the right quality, even if you feel on the back foot after a tenuous introduction – because this first deal will set a precedent.

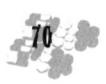

Ideally your first bag should be of the highest quality: grams on the generous side, no dud pills, maybe even the odd freebie to get you reeled in (a real playground trick).

Dealers hold junkies and rich-kids in equal contempt as much as all junkies and rich-kids think dealers are scumbags.

MUTUAL RESPECT IS NOT THE ISSUE HERE; BUSINESS IS.

After all, it may not feel like it when making desperate phonecalls at 4am, but don't forget it's a buyer's market. Your dealer should care about customer satisfaction.

Giving you a good deal early on is like the dealer's loyalty card scheme, to make sure you call him first up next time you're drunk.

Any dealer who feels he can skank you first time around doesn't want to make a second deal. Quite probably he's the guy you just met in the street or in a minicab, he's offloading some loss-making product and he won't have any more in the coffers for the future... maybe he only had chewing gum, soap-bar and baking soda in the first place.

Such people are not the contacts worth cultivating, socially or commercially. A man with a reliable supply and a steady business will always feather the beds with new clients, however small-fry.

Remember, it's the little deals that add up, the little people that count in this business.

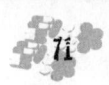

However much a dealer makes on a big night, he's never too proud to turn down a little more.

Call him late at night. Call him first thing in the morning. Call him on a Sunday or a weeknight... only on Xmas Day or when he has been arrested will his mobile be switched off

Think corporate: Demand More! Expect The Best! He'll come running, and hiding his smirk while he does.

Mobile phones have revolutionised the drug market. Now they can be ordered like takeaway – one guy has the number while everyone else shouts their order round the table.

'Three horse bhunas. A skunk baghee. A hashwari naan. And get him to throw some poppadums in.'

Rumours used to be told of New York's 'special' taxi service, which delivered to your door 24/7 no questions asked... well, post 'Cool Britannia' and the New Deal, Britain's major cities expect just the same.

Cultivate the right people, skulk along to enough shady deals and sit meekly in the back seat of enough Beamers and pretty soon your phone book will be filling up with unlikely, self-parodying names.

You'll need to file them in their own caller group marked 'Dealers' or (more subtly) **'Meals on Wheels'**.

Names like Ibiza Paul and Irish Mike; Crazy John and King B; Corsa, Caballero, French Toni and Fast Eddie.

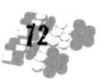

Some of them will be named after their cars, others their country of origin. These are both usually untruths: chances are **'Maltese Steve'** comes from Leeds and **'Mercedes'** drives a Mondeo. Like call-girls, they know the value of sounding exotic.

Enjoy the range of options while they last; once you've been in the game for a while you'll notice a pretty high turnover of arrests and busts in the big cities.

The wise dealers will change their number every 6 months, so it's a case of 'Use it or Lose it'; the unwise end up in prison. It's sad, the way you and a favourite contact can just, you know, drift apart. Remember, you are under no obligation to visit him in prison.

Generally when they get greedy they get caught. They couldn't just retire at the magic figure, that dream vehicle, the ceiling they set themselves five years before when they'd get out of the game.

They had to cling on for more, that even more ostentatious car. When you see that Porsche, when they start boasting, then showing you the 10kg concrete slabs marked with the 'prancing horse' logo of the Ferrari cartel, well, it's time to find a new dealer.

In this incorruptible country where dealers don't run the economy and politicians can't be bought, that's probably as big as they'll be allowed to get without becoming a respected entrepreneur and Labour Party donor.

How to do Drugs

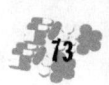

Don't worry, the fuzz aren't interested in the little fish like you. Once they've nailed the source they won't chase up every number in their phone records; and even if they did there's a Hippocratic oath all dealers have to sign at drug school to protect client confidentiality. And don't feel guilty either, **'Big Ali'** knew the risk.

When dialling a new dealer, remember this simple introductory phrase. 'Hey, is that Juan? Yo Spanish, it's John. Yeah, you remember me, I'm a mate of John's. Yeah John, from John's party. Doing good... Look, are you anywhere near Richmond?'

NB If by chance you don't know anyone who buys or takes drugs, so you can't get even get a foot in the door, then frankly don't get started.

They're no fun to do on your own in a one-horse town, and throwing yourself in at the deep end in Glasgow or Brixton will most likely see you killed.

Plus, if you really don't know ANYONE then you're probably either too young to try it, too old to risk it... or too boring for it to make any difference.

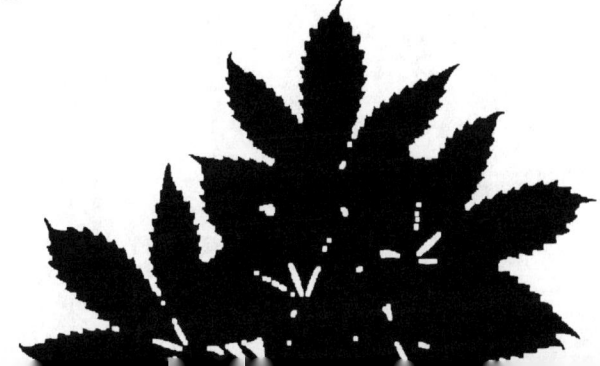

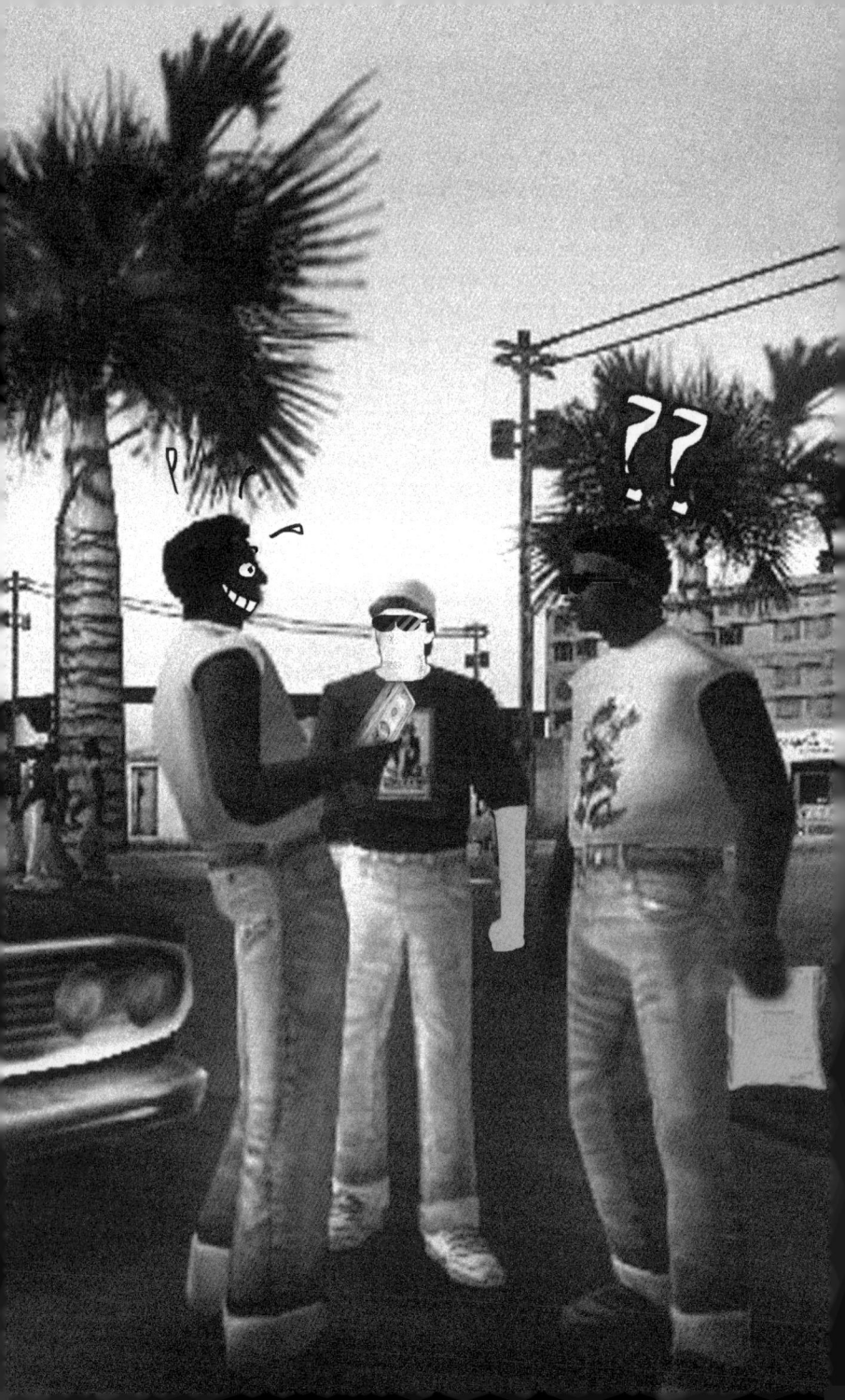

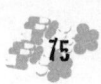

STREET SCORING

Ah, now this is a different game altogether, with a high chance of being skanked, mugged or bum-raped. Once upon a time all drug deals were done like this... so many problems.

> Who do you trust?
> Is it safer to ask or wait to be approached?
> Do you hand over the cash first or try to get the product first?

The answer is, you're totally unsafe.

You play it by ear on the basis that you trust no-one but eventually you're going to have to hand over some cash, otherwise you've wasted half an hour talking to one of the most unpleasant people you've ever met.

Alternately he and his friends might turn nasty, in which case your evening could end on the operating table of your nearest infirmary.

As you banter and jostle you must try to work yourself into a position of respect – whilst aware of the huge irony of that word in the context of pathetically begging for dirty highs off lowlife who scare the shit out of you.

**Don't act too cool:
he wants to be taken seriously.**

**Don't act too scared:
he'll eat you for breakfast.
Slip him the notes too obviously and you
will unnerve and irritate him.**

Act too paranoid or surreptitious and you will irritate and unnerve him.

Remember, these guys watch the same movies as you – go for the time-honoured **Goodfellows** manoeuvres.

Look over your shoulder and push the folding money in his hand in the same drop of the shoulders.

If you're lucky he will drop something in your left hand as you do this, but there's no time to check as doing this right means doing it quickly.

Once you've inspected it you may realise a number of things.

That he has spat chewing gum in your hand. That he has wrapped up foil in some more foil and rolled it in a ball. That he has given you a half of speed instead of a gram of coke, a bit of gravel instead of some crack.

Comfort yourself with the thought that even if he had given you what you'd asked for you'd still have been wasting your money.

Take it home, rack it up and talk shit anyway.

Crush a tin can and smoke the ash and aluminium fumes. Face it, you only bought it to give yourself something to do or else you'd already have a proper reputable dealer and wouldn't need this book.

How to do Drugs

In the unlikely event that you got what you paid for, maybe you managed to convince him you meant business.

Maybe he thought you'd be back, or he swallowed it when you assured him that if his stuff was good you'd be regular (and in the case of most of those laxative white powders, you'd be right). Or maybe he just felt sorry for you. Either way, don't automatically expect to do so well next time. You haven't cracked it, just got lucky.

SCORING OFF TRAMPS

Often, a man lying in a bag on the side of a street will know the haunts of every dealer in the district.

> **TOP TIP** Get a friend to do the talking, and promise to back him up if it gets nasty. Of course, just in case it DOES get nasty be planning an escape route as he haggles, not letting anyone block you off down a subway or alley. If this shifty behaviour spooks the dealers, get out of there early.
> I'm sure your pal will understand, eventually.

> **TOP DON'T** Making jokes about being undercover policemen. You know how customs hate the old line about declaring 'only the crown jewels'? Well, custom officials don't carry blades. Of course, dealers are naturally suspicious. If they test their own produce, they're naturally paranoid too. Ride with the constant suspicious eyes and doubletalk, and join in with any good-natured cop-killing banter.

But don't accept offers from gentlemen of the road to be your 'go-between' if you want to see your money put to good use... except maybe by the tramp himself.

Obviously in the great chain of command there are going to be middle-men between you and the Medellin cartel inflating the price, but keep them to a minimum.

When you're paying a tramp in Soho to go off and find his regular brown dealer you shouldn't hold your breath, not unless you've retained his dog on a string for security.

Even if he honestly meant to help you out he's still prone to forgetfully wandering round the block singing to strangers instead of tracking down his man.

If you want any success choose a tramp who you pass by every day coming back from work, so he knows you know where he lives, or rather doesn't.

Then he might start seeing you as a regular guy to sting for a tenner if he gets it right. Also, offering to share the hit shows good faith, and further discourages your new friend from slipping you wrapfuls of domestic cleaner.

HOWEVER THIS KIND OF RELATIONSHIP DOES NO GOOD FOR THE SELF-ESTEEM OF EITHER PARTY, SO DON'T SHIT TOO CLOSE TO YOUR OWN DOORSTEP.

SCORING IN A FOREIGN COUNTRY

This sounds like an advanced skill, but often this can be easier and certainly more pleasant than in some shitty Bristolian hole or dark dive in Leeds. At least you have the weather and warm evenings when scouting around for a holiday hit.

People are just as dishonest, sure, but you expect them to be: you're English, you're a xenophobe, you're automatically on your guard.

You may not speak their language but the great thing about being English is, they probably speak yours. They will also speak the universal lingua franca – the language of money – better than you.

All you really need to be aware of is:

a)   Are you in a country that violently disapproves of drugs, be it for religious or public morality reasons? If so, be careful who you start asking. A citizen's arrest might be followed by a twenty stretch in a Phuket jail (see also 'Smuggling').

b)   Are you in a country where simply being an English tourist carrying money means you might get mugged, stripped and thrown in a ditch? These might include Columbia and Scotland.

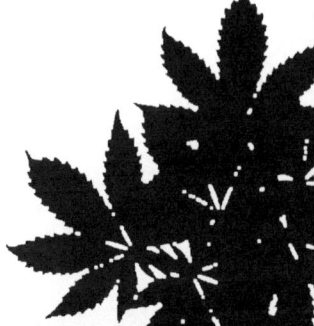

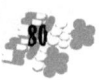

In the latter case, be careful who you agree to go down a dark alley with clutching fifty notes. Make sure you're with visible friends who know where you're going, or at least alert the British Consulate that you're off to buy drugs with a tall man in a fez.

Life can be cheap in some places, especially the life of a no-good junkie like yourself. They'd probably slot your throat for the blackmarket trade in human organs, if only your liver was in better shape.

If you've made sure of these things then be bold, ask away: chances are you're in a Mediterranean holiday town and English-speaking dealers from miles around have moved there to make it big and retire young.

Sit at a bar near the centre and eye up every passer-by as a potential score, much as you might eye up the senoritas and/or dusky moustachioed waiters were you a mere civilian.

Nudge your friend if a pale, thin-looking scrag limps over, or a big fattie in a gold tracksuit grunts by on a moped, and drool: 'Phwoar, Look at the drugs on that!'

Remember, holidays are about experimentation. Try something new. You don't go to Spain and order fish'n'chips every night, do you? **(Well, you might, but then you're not the sort of cultured person we want reading this book).**

Be adventurous and let some exotic tastes into your life – stuff you might turn your nose up at were it just a rainy Tuesday night in Islington.

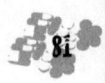

Your dad's just had another sherry, your nan's let herself have that cigarette...

Try some 'dirty'. You're on holiday, it doesn't count.

If you're still worried about the language barrier, then the inevitable 'English-style' pubs/sports bars in central city districts are probably as good as anywhere to make discreet enquiries (again, though, steer clear of anyone who looks too Combat 18 – some of these ex-pat bartenders are further right than Franco).

Not only can they serve you a bacon buttie and lager in pints, you can also speak to someone you actually understand – although the quality and value will probably be lower (that goes for both drugs and conversation).

Really, it's just like home from home. In fact you might as well have hung out around Yates' Wine Lodge back in Colchester for a fortnight.

Certain other countries, however, have quirks that actually make your life easier – opium dens still operating in Vietnam, coke in South America that's so cheap they use it to line the beaches, wild mushrooms harvested fresh in Mexico, the drug-crazed loved-up Burning Man festival in Nevada.

The obvious example closer to home (excepting the likes of Dublin, Glasgow and Edinburgh, European Cities of Scag) is Amsterdam. But make it quick: **the locals are finally getting bored of the endless stag weekends and 3-day benders and are lobbying**

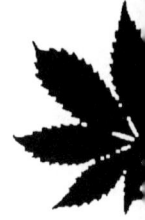

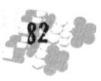

to have things like laws reintroduced.

Less well-known than Amsterdam, but enjoying many of the same legal laxities and loopholes, is Zurich: a beautiful place to buy packs of freeze-dried mushrooms with funny instructions from high-street psychedelia shops **(sample content: 'the user may experience sensation of being paint or box of chips')**.

TOP TIP Don't pay more than a tenner for a wrap of shouting powder in Rio, even in tourist spots.
Save the rest for a helicopter ride or going to the Maracena stadium or learning to scuba dive or something CIVILISED.

TOP DON'T Don't think that by finding cheaper drugs, you should expect to be saving money on a night out. Instead simply buy six times as much cocaine as you would back in England.
Then at 5am, instead of having to call up reinforcements, spend your back-up budget on some toothless hooker who'd give you a terrible disease if only you had the slightest chance of actually getting it up.

How to do Drugs

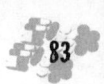

Holland in particular is full of these tourist-traps, where you can buy all the necessary paraphernalia (see, er, 'paraphernalia'), herbal alternatives, viagra, amyl, and a wide menu with all flavours of dope and hallucinogens.

All very well, but frankly boring when it's all above board.

These gimmicky places are however excellent spots, when the coast is clear of other customers, to start asking about where the real stuff is kept.

They may not have it under the counter, but they might meet you round the back – or draw you a helpful diagram to a nearby bar with a scribbled reference and the name of a guy to ask for. Easy.

To find these Info Centres for Drug Tourists, just look for the lava lamps in the window and the rainbow-beads instead of doors.

SCORING BY MAIL-ORDER

Oh, so you've seen those mail-order ads in the back of subculture magazines, have you?

**Herbal E's and real hemp plants available by post? By all means, send off.
It's only money.**

> **Why not get a pump-action penis extender while you're at it?**
>
> **Some pheromone spray made of cats' piss to make you more attractive to the opposite sex?**
>
> **Be sure to leave your full details so they can send them on to their 'colleagues' to let you know about other exciting rip-offs.**

As a matter of fact there were changes in the law a few years back that mean you can get 'real' soft drugs by mail, depending on the way they were prepared (or, legally speaking, 'not' prepared).

We're talking buds and seeds instead of resin, mushrooms that have only dried naturally in the jiffy bag, that sort of thing.

The difficulty is identifying the bona fide organisations.

You want names and addresses?

What do you think this is, the Rough Guide?

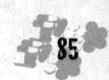

Frankly if you're not prepared to invest more than the price of a stamp in making your score then you don't deserve this book.

> I'm more interested in people for whom the phrases 'REAL soft drugs' makes them uncomfortable.

FINALLY...
A DRUG TOUR OF GLASGOW

Not enough room here, that's really a whole other book...

A quick dishonourable mention to the natives' drug of choice, however – **'Bucky'**.

It's short for Buckfast Tonic Wine, a bizarre and undrinkable slop brewed by a group of eccentric monks in Devon. The monks themselves are teetotal, which is understandable once you taste it. So strongly do locals feel about the stuff that nearby pubs refuse to stock it – in fact the council insists it be taken as far away from Devon as international trade ethics permit. Hence nearly all of it ends up in Scotland, where it is greedily downed by tramps.

Each sizzling bottle is accompanied by the sobering warning that 'the word tonic is in no way intended to indicate any medicinal properties whatsoever'. In that sense, it is truly a drug worthy of the name.

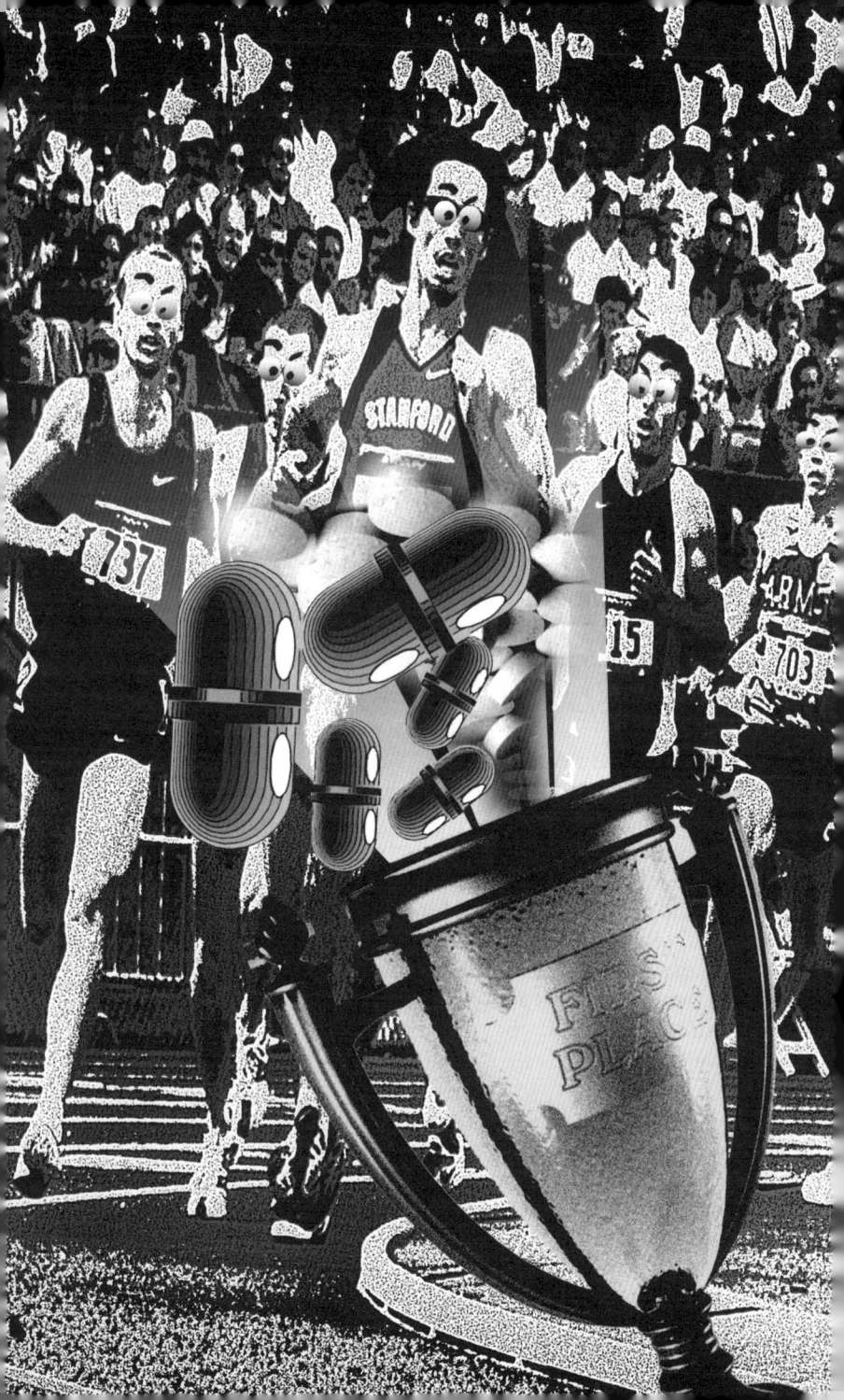

It seems ironic that drugs and sports are only really associated together in terms of cheating and performance enhancement, as all my experiences point directly to the contrary.

Real drugs do not assist a healthy lifestyle or improve your co-ordination – not any of the good ones, anyway.

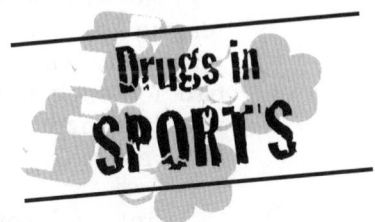

RECREATIONAL ('A BIT OF FUN')

The defining image of recreational drug use in sport dates from the 1994 World Cup, when Diego Maradona announced his short-lived comeback with a great goal – and a frenzied, wide-eyed, coke-fuelled gurn at the camera.

That would have been the moment when someone thought it might be a good idea to swab his piss, just to be on the safe side.

Some of our own most treasured footballers resent the suggestion that as young men in their 20s earning £50k a week, they might be partial to the odd nose-up.

But the idea that cocaine helps rather than hinders their performances seems laughable; if you want an energy kick (not to mention fizzy piss) take a Lucozade tablet.

Generally, soft drugs and sport only go together in events where you'd choke if you ever heard a commentator

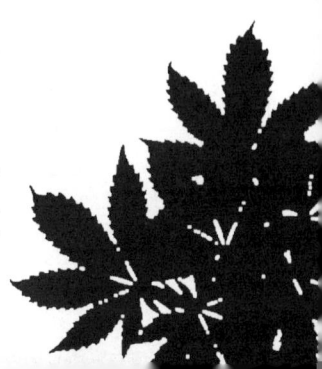

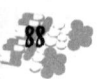

use the word 'athlete' – hairy, lazy English cricketers for example, or beer-bellied darts players.

You will occasionally hear of a lower-league or Conference footballer testing positive for cannabis, but what's the point in a ban for such nobodies? Being laid-back and wholly unmotivated is no leg-up in professional sport.

Drink is even worse, as anyone who's warmed up for Sunday League at a pub can tell you. But after some quite fun research, I can reveal that after staying up all night caning it on Saturday, a bit of fresh air can give you second wind.

Pills and dancing take it out on the legs, but they're better for your game than the booze culture that still poisons the breath of our national sport.

> **When 'returning to fitness', Paul Gascoigne was once photographed enjoying a pint of Guinness on the training pitch.**
> Incidentally, he once charmingly described his black England team-mate Paul Ince as 'looking like a pint of Guinness' when he bravely played on with the top of his head wrapped in a white bandage.
> But then a lot of people get a bit racist after a few drinks.

NON-RECREATIONAL ('CHEATING')

Steroids, stimulants and male hormones: these are where drugs and sports REALLY fall out. As such substances have no great recreational value (except to the very vain – gym-bunnies, bodybuilders and transsexuals) then there's little reason to give them time of day in these pages, except to ask the question: what is actually wrong with it?

> If sport is entertainment, then coaches have a right, in fact a duty, to see how fast we can possibly make a human being go (providing the public can watch).

Pumping a consenting adult full of Billy Whizz till he nearly pops? Winding him up then watching how he goes? It should be done in the name of science AND getting bums on seats.

How can an athlete in good conscience say he has given his all, pushed his body to the limit of human endurance, until he has tried saturating his bloodstream with rocket fuel?

After all, most clubbers and caners push their bodies to the dark limits of human endurance week in week out, and we don't get medals. Ordinary fuckheads pull off medical miracles every Saturday night, without the money or public adulation reserved for our pampered, overpaid athletes.

The system is already unfair, with richer countries better able to cover up the traces of their, ahem, 'dietary' regimes.

We won't get a level playing field till every man jack is allowed to try the same shit before the big race.

Anyway, not so long ago they called it unsportsmanlike even to gain advantage over an opponent by bothering to train.

Have top boffins at the British Library struck the works of Huxley or Coleridge from the literary canon because they were achieved only under the influence of mind-expanding substances?

Did the Supreme Court undo Clinton's reformist agenda, burn the profits of his economic policy, because his progressive social ideas were first conceived while stoned in a campus bedsit, then pushed through on a cocaine-induced high of self-validation?

Hell no!

But this is only the same principle in force when we deny near-superhuman sprint times entry to the record books, on some mere technicality like steroid use or a course of human growth hormone.

Hilary and Tensing were artificially assisted by oxygen when they hit the summit of Everest, and Churchill was drunk when he gave most of his speeches: these are just the performance-enhancing drugs that society let through the net.

I say, reinstate Ben Johnson's 100m win at the 1988 Olympics and give that British Olympic skier his bronze back – all he did was have a Lemsip because it was bloody brass monkeys, and if it was chilly on the slopes I'd do the same.

Incidentally, Ben's time may have finally been broken 'legitimately' - that's to say, by cleverer drug cheats. But try to run in a straight line next time YOU'RE tanked up, and if you make it anywhere like 100m I'll give you a medal myself. That's a measure of the man's achievement in 1988.

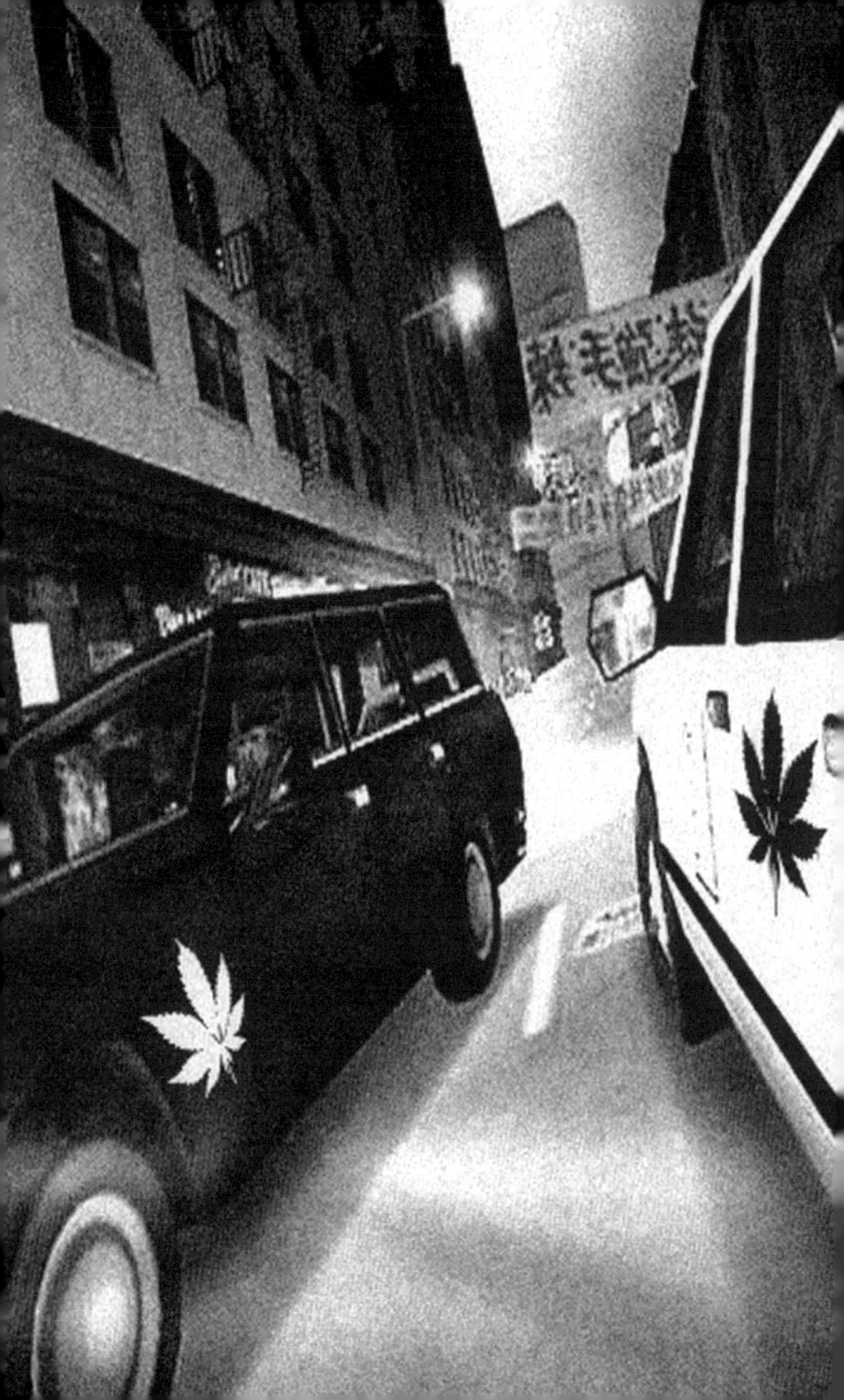

DRINK 'n' DRIVE: Everyone knows this is strictly illegal, and generally unwise.

However, the law has provision for a certain degree of alcoholic intake behind the wheel – indeed such measures actively encourage drivers to fulfil their legal allocation, else look like a flake in the eyes of their peers.

Working on the (utterly misleading) assumption that alcohol is just another drug that 'they' forgot to ban, we can assume in a fair and equal world that there would be an acceptable limit apportioned to ANY mind-altering substance beneath which one was still capable in the eyes of the law.

Drugs and DRIVING

There would also be narcotic-free alternatives available for the designated driver in any shop or street corner, for example wraps of talcum powder, bags of cooking herbs or plain blotting paper, so the unlucky designate wouldn't have to miss out on the social side of the activity while ferrying his mates about.

Here are the recommended limits for drug intake behind the wheel.

Please bear in mind they are not yet endorsed by the DVLA or Highway Police, and are applicable on a strictly self-regulatory basis answerable to the individual conscience.

This does not constitute a legal defence.

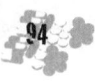

Marijuana

Some drivers maintain they operate better with a joint, becoming calmer and more thoughtful drivers (not to mention considerate – 'road rage' incidents, for instance, become particularly uncommon amongst the medicinally mellow).

However, as ever with users there is a strong element of self-delusion going on here. Chugging along behind the wheel in an unhurried bubble of your own, treating the world as your slow lane – such behaviour is rightly considered a menace to other road users when perpetrated by the old, blind and doddery.

Why should the young and stoned feel superior exhibiting the same road manner, just because they've got ragga whacked up on the stereo?

Equally those behind-the-wheel decisions may seem more considered, but the simple reason for this is they are actually taking much longer: an average of 2-3 seconds longer pondering the philosophical truth of lane-choosing, or whether to avoid the child on the zebra crossing.

Do I steer into the skid or out of it? Does red mean stop or go, and what does it mean when the car behind has flashing blue lights?

These questions seem far less pressing after a smoke, but sometimes urgency of thought is a necessary evil. Unlike most of the vacuous philosophical crap that flashes through your 'expanded' mind, these apparently mundane road-safety issues are actually MORE important in real life than they seem to be when you're stoned.

On the plus side, increasingly lax cannabis laws are encouraging more and more drivers to wind down their windows on a sunny day to enjoy a pre-rolled one-y ('single dose joint'); and as more road-users also become 'users', the more likely they are to share the same time-delay in indicating, steering and braking.

Remember, keeping an open window or sunroof means your vehicle is less likely to turn itself into a giant bong – which can be a good or a bad thing. It depends on whether you're parked in a field staring at the stars or travelling up the M1.

Overall, a mild smoke is unlikely to do any harm. Skunk yourself into a stupor, however, and you will deserve any paranoid freak-out that may hit you when there's a firm tap at the window and a sniffy policeman asks why you've failed to move at the lights for ten minutes.

> Suggested limit
> One for the road

Cocaine

Ah, the old tiger in your tank. Generally one of the safer modes of illegal driving, and recommended to take the edge off alcohol.

However, if one of the stated evils of drunk-driving is 'artificially increased confidence', then you can be sure it applies double to Charlie. Use in moderation.

Chief problem is how to take it at the wheel.

A bullet (see Paraphernalia) is thus convenient for a shot in the arm, so to speak, when on long journeys (remember the slogan, Tiredness Can Kill).

A passenger is helpful for preparation of the chamber. Otherwise you require at least two passengers: one to rack up and hold the CD case, road atlas or whatever, and the other to hold the wheel and/or gearstick while you take hands and eyes off the road to do the nostril housework.

Careful, sudden braking while a rolled fifty is lodged up your nose can be very dangerous (although frankly a bloody pinky rammed into your brain is probably the least you deserve considering the risks you're taking with everybody else's lives).

Suggested limit
2–3 hits. But don't cross too many white lines.

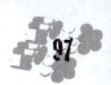

Ecstasy

Not recommended at all. If you plan to drop before driving, make sure your journey is less than thirty minutes long and does not require a return leg.

If you start to come up, obey the Think! Road Safety signs and pull over into the hard shoulder for a responsible period of recollection, remembering at all times to turn up the cheesy house anthems and wave your arms in the air until safe to proceed. This may be several hours.

Suggested limit
Journeys under half an hour, tops.

Hallucinogenics

**Absolutely out of the question.
Unfortunately flashbacks while at the wheel are always a possibility.**

The only relevant experiences my students have shared with me were characterised by criminality and mortal fear, although they are stories worth telling the grandchildren.

One involved a big bag of mushrooms and what appeared to be a police tail, which required an escape plan so brave and stupid it meant turning up a stranger's drive and parking in his garage at 1am.

So that the cop car would eventually decide the driver had made it safely home, the passengers brazenly had to let themselves in at the back door and make a cup of tea. Two hours squatting on a darkened kitchen later, they left a thank-you note for the hospitality and continued safely on their journey.

Another patient was spiked with three drops of liquid LSD, and came round in a car with a gun held to his head and the accusation of being a suicide bomber.

Apparently he'd decided he wasn't fit to drive and decided to park somewhere secluded off road – which turned out to be the Israeli embassy. The scariest thing, he claimed, was having to drive off again.

Suggested limit
Try none at all.

Speed

How does this affect your driving?
The answer's in the question.

Suggested use
Not in built-up areas with speed bumps.

Viagra

Now this I've not tried.
It doesn't sound like a particularly clever idea, but
that's not to say it's not worth doing.

Beware confusion when operating the gearstick, however. It can also very difficult to see off an erection while driving on your own, so invite along a friend in the passenger seat. Just make sure they're a very good friend.

Suggested use
For long, hard journeys.

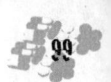

Heroin

This author has no driving experience on the drug whatsoever to report. Generally, actually getting somewhere is not what tends to be at the forefront of one's mind on heroin.

Suggested use
None, but sell your car. You'll be needing the cash soon enough.

Dealing with the Old Bill

These are the same rules you'd apply when pulled over for any driving offence: turn on a sunny face, show them the deference they crave, and your chances of not being stop-searched – or in some way willfully inconvenienced – improve radically. If you have harder drugs on you it may require a substantial contribution to the old Policeman's Ball (tuck a rolled-up fifty into the licence wallet when you hand over your details).

Traditionally, it does also help to be white in these situations. However, post-Macpherson report, it has become easy to play on their fears if you are darker than they are. Remind them that they have stop-and-search quotas for white guys in nice cars too, and intimate strongly that you may have an undercover film-crew in your boot. Whatever your colour, the cheekiness and near-the-knuckle nature of your banter should be weighed against the sheer quantity of drugs about your person. By all means crack a gentle gag about getting home before the munchies kick in, but don't push it if you're packing some of Colombia's national treasure.

REMEMBER: The petty social inadequate knocking at your window joined the force to get the sense of self- importance and respect that no-one would give him in real life. Be charming and polite but try not to give him an inch.

Food is one of life's more indulgent pleasures, and its preparation considered a noble art – likewise society revels in the ceremony of doing it socially.

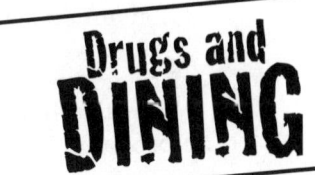

Drugs and DINING

Yet despite these similarities to drug use the two are not generally well mixed, and drug consumption can disrupt healthy eating patterns quite considerably. And vice versa.

What's more, some might consider your drug use insensitive if preparing you a nice meal.

Most obvious are the extremes of smoke and coke. We'll start with the marijuana.

The 'munchies' is a phenomenon widely documented. However, while smoking spliff clearly has the potential to unlock one's appetite, the process is not instant.
Light up before dinner, and chances are you'll just toy with your evening meal talking shit then come bedtime be overcome with the kind of hunger pangs that only a spell in Auschwitz could induce.

This is why you end up round the corner in the rain trying to locate a 24-hour garage. This is why you find yourself there at 2am buying Ginsters and biscuits in unnecessary quantities so you can use your credit card.

This is why crisp bags and Twix wrappers will fill your ashtrays when you come to clear up in the morning.

How to do Drugs

In short, it's a poor diet: there's a reason why students and crusties look so pasty-faced.

The dark mistress 'munchies' will crave convenience foods at inconvenient times. If you have no access to junk food you may even be motivated to start cooking late into the night, when least capable of doing so, most probably in somebody else's kitchen.

Not only is this an insult to your host, it is also a recipe for mishap. Take this eyewitness account, from a Mr B. of Chester:

> 'Recently I tried to cook a midnight Mariner's Pie after a desperate, dope-addled raid on the freezer. I didn't really take the packet instructions very seriously, partly because I couldn't really get to grips with what they were asking of me. Preheat the oven? Why wait? 40 minutes at 200 degrees?
>
> But the passing of time has no meaning! A quick stretch on the sofa later and I decided it would probably be ready. There it was, frozen in the middle, dangerously lukewarm around the edges, just a big shellfish gloop topped in a mix of processed potato and melted plastic from where I'd failed to peel off the packaging. I wolfed it down and, needless to say, was sick as a dog the next day.'

Actually it's amazing what your body can take in its stride sometimes, when immunised from taste or fear or pain by a shedload of narcotics, but it's best not to take the risk and just go to bed hungry.

Remember, your metabolism is worst at digesting when you're asleep, even more so comatose. Don't eat shit last thing at night, pass out and then complain about bloating and wind in the morning. You'll get no sympathy from me or your bedpartner, unless you are both into... well we won't explore that.

Coke is a different beast: the unsociable killer of many a dinner party. Think before you get your nose down; it's an after-dinner mint, not something to tickle the tastebuds between courses like a sorbet or a cigarette. It clears the palette, sure, but it wipes out the appetite as well.

Nevertheless, the cocaine age is still raging. Statistically, someone will be packing snow at your dinner party, and it might as well be you.

Just remember modern times require modern manners. As a rule of thumb, don't start to chop lines if there are still plates and crap on the table. Wait for the table to be cleared: this is a sign that you may rack up freely now that the main meal is out of the way. Beware of the sudden laxative effect though – some dealers are unmindful of Health & Safety guidelines when they cut their charlie.

> **ONE FINAL CULINARY TIP WITH CHARLIE**
> Try and save a little for breakfast. You may find it helps a lot getting the day started (if your sensitive nostrils can brook it). And if you're prone to an acid tummy, stock up on Pepto-Bismol.

Other drugs have different quirks.

Speed is historically favoured by the modelling industry; just like coke it's an appetite suppressant, but it's not full of all that high-calorie nutritional goodness that can make for 'coke fatties'.

Heroin is famous for making you throw up, hence pointless to combine with a square meal.

And lysergic elements can twist all kinds of awkward knots in your stomach, rendering the whole digestive process a nightmare 3D fun-ride though your alimentary canal.

Another top tip on balancing your drugs diet: when it comes to hallucinogenics, certain edibles will take the edge off, so steer clear of citric fruits, sugar and vitamin C if it's a full-on trip you're after.

Alternatively, DO seek them out if you want to get back on top of the situation.

For the true gourmand, a quick note on mixing drugs: treat them like jellybeans, delicious on their own, but exciting to create new flavours by combination.

Some contradict each other, some compliment; coke takes the edge off E, dope does strange things to the acid mind. Try it yourself and see. Above all, as with cooking: experiment!

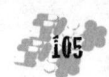

"It provokes the desire
but it takes away the performance..."
(Macbeth Act 2, Sc iii)

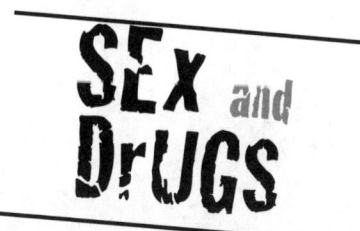

So Shakespeare's Porter described the experience of mixing ecstasy and coke.

Sex and Drugs are not always the natural combination the glamour cliché implies. For gentlemen, Coke is a no-no if you're expected to perform, even if the swagger in your step has made you more attractive to the opposite sex (or so you thought).

Beware one-night stands forged on this drug: they may indeed last a whole night but your trouser credentials may not be shown to best advantage.

'You ever fucked on cocaine Mick?' **purrs Sharon Stone inanely in Basic Instinct.** 'It feels nice.'

And well she might think so, all she has to do is lay back and think of England (well, in her case, America but it's not the same). The average man, on the other hand, will spend most of the night trying to 'thumb in' his slackened member, grimacing as his frustrated partner attempts to invigorate the shrivelled shrimp with fist or teeth.

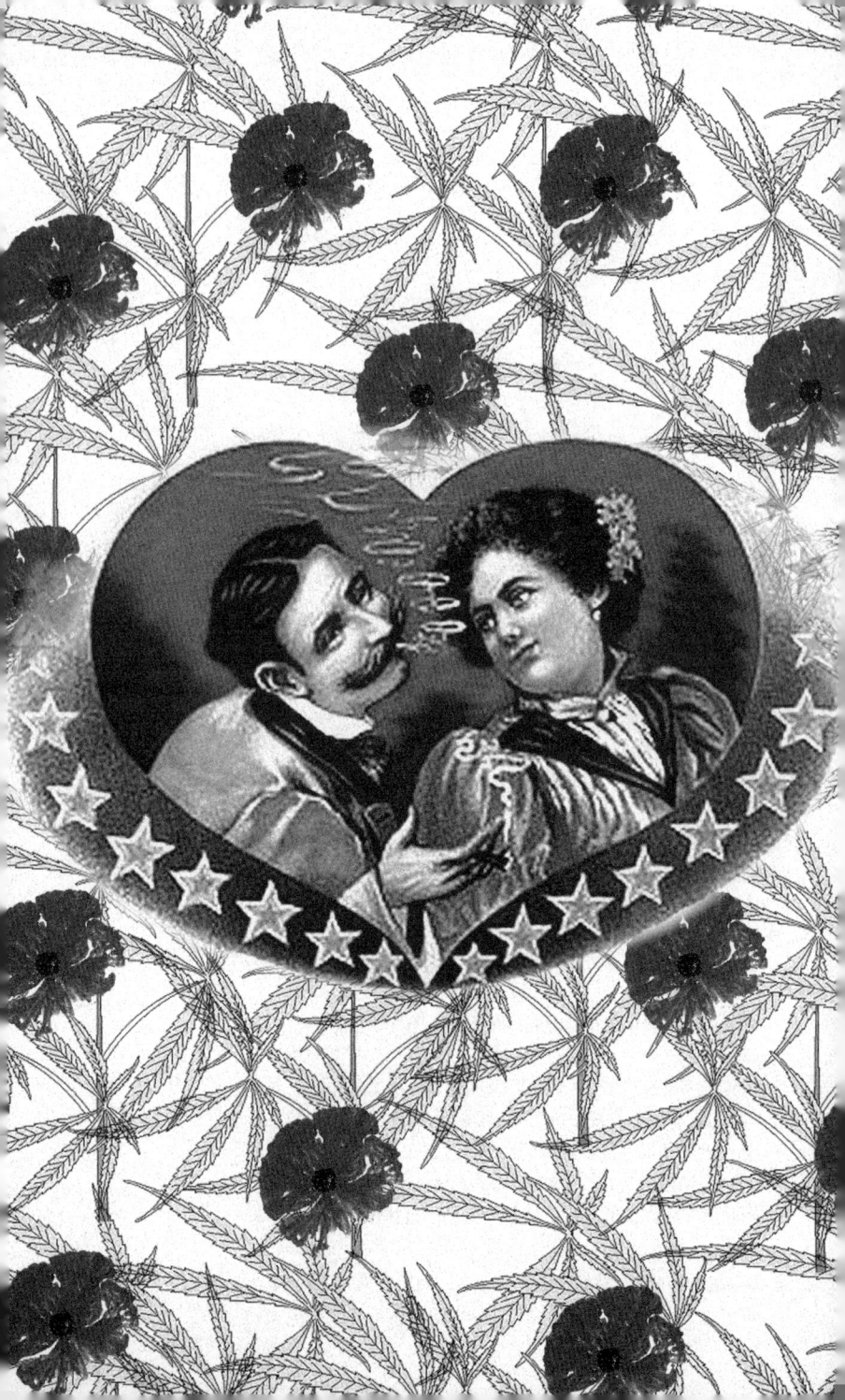

Of course, it's not all bad. Toot can be a boon to the man who suffers from premature ejaculation: indeed it is readily endorsed by GPs to save the blushes of the hyper-sensitive, whether ingested or simply rubbed in like talcum.

Some girls may claim they enjoy an intimate application, though most soon find this scuppers their slim chances of achieving a result.

Still, power is an aphrodisiac, and coke is power: essentially, it's extract of money in its most purified form. Certainly the odd line can be used seductively (perhaps 'off the tits', the seedy hotel-room classic, or out of the inner thigh if the bone definition is good enough); used moderately, it's the perfect set-up for a lovemaking session to last two or even three hours.

Tantric sex without the yoga, you might even say. But it's those long, boozy, jaw-champing nights of marathon nose abuse that leave a man shrivelled and his woman impatient.

Worst of all, if you go home alone, and find yourself lying in bed unable to drift off, your instinct may lead you to onanism.
A terrible thought.

If you finally succeed in the futile, long-drawn-out grapple... well, it might just about release enough soporific endorphins to let you pass out, but come the morning you'll be red-raw and very sore.

Viagra is a consideration by way of antidote. Although designed for limp old men and drooping soaks who need a litre of scotch even to look at the wife, young loving couples can use the same stuff to counteract the effects of cocaine.

However, the decision to take it is one you need to make pretty early in the evening, as all the coke will slow the process down.

If you're on the singles scene, it helps to be certain you're going to get lucky before dropping the expensive little bastard, or you'll have a lot of explaining to do when you wake up with an unsightly tent-pole in someone's front room.

Even when you pull, the coke/Viagra cocktail can give you the worst of both worlds: a no-show when it matters then a raging bonk-on long after the bird has flown. This can last all through the next morning at work, when embarrassingly surrounded by guys in suits or topless builders (depending on your line of work).

> No amount of sneaky 'toilet breaks' will sort you out before lunchtime.

For similar reasons beware trying your first as a drunken late-night prank.

A surprising number of secretly curious men first taste it this way, go to bed complaining it doesn't work on REAL men, then wake up at a peculiar angle unable to get their trousers on.

> Oh – and girls, remember the flipside to this artificial erection business:
> **just because it's up doesn't always mean it's interested.**

That's right, six hours of stiffness in bed with a woman can be less fun (and more painful) for blokes than it sounds. It can't completely solve age-old marital problems like whether you actually fancy your wife anymore.

Equally, she may not appreciate loving post-coital cuddles that poke her in the ribs all night. Key phrases you'll both need to learn to be diplomatic to your partner: 'Get off, that hurts' and 'I'm trying to sleep'.

Mind you, no drugs are an exact science and the effects are different for different people. For women especially (who I consider more different than most) the experiences range from sustained and intensified orgasmic excitement to absolutely fuck all effect.

Some of the so-called testimonials of women 'loving it' on Viagra can be discounted on the basis that the entire sex are a bunch of untrustworthy liars and fakers anyway.

More reliably, a gentleman will usually find an effect on his 'gentleman' with a 25-50mg dose. Just make sure you feel the benefit at a time when it isn't ragingly inconvenient.

There are less clinical alternatives in the chemical world. But just because ecstasy is a 'love drug' doesn't mean it's properly medicinal, nor is it likely to make you a smooth-talker.

More likely you'll become a jabbering nincompoop with wide eyes and a grinding jaw... but fortunately so will everybody else and it won't stop you finding them appealing.

Be careful not to confuse affection with sexual attraction, though, or to confuse anyone else. You may suddenly realise everyone in the room is your 'best friend', but that still doesn't mean it's wise to buddy-fuck.

Above all make sure you don't inflict these sweaty, over-amorous moves on anyone NOT in something approaching the same state.

TOP TIP:
If they are as high as you, look out for

a) Best friends,
b) Best friends' girlfriends or boyfriends,
c) People of the wrong gender
(according to preference)
and
d) Family members.

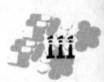

THE 'SUMMER OF LOVE' MYTH

Strange to think in the '60s what they called the 'Summer of Love' was all about joints and acid. What unlikely bedroom companions they now seem.

Lighting up a joint in bed can only mean it's time to sleep, then there's the risk of hot rocks on the nice valance.

As for LSD... there's no telling what it'll do to your partner's looks.

You might get three breasts, you might start seeing varicose veins moving like snakes, or you just might find yourself in bed with Grotbags or the child-catcher from Chitty Chitty Bang Bang.

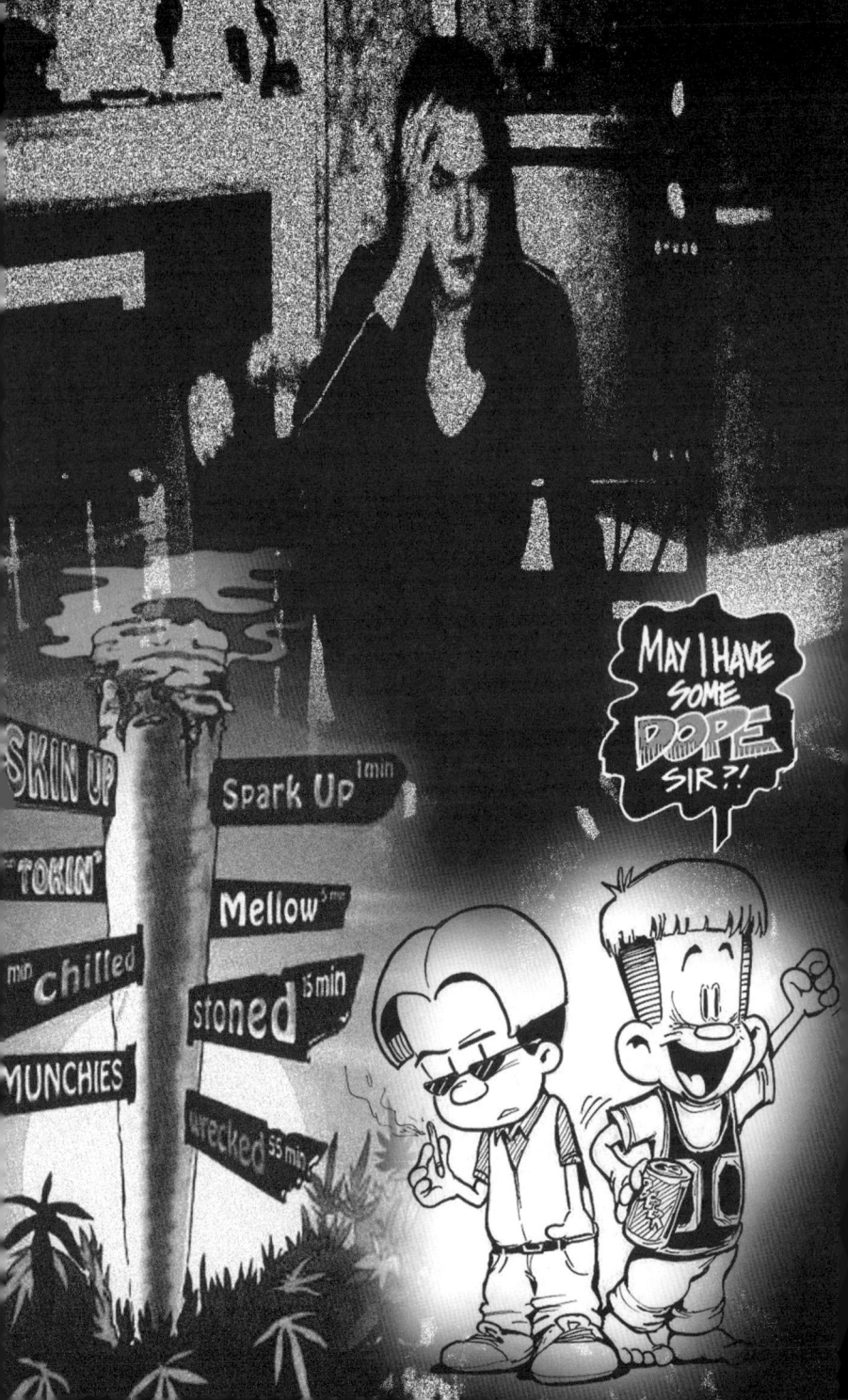

Notes for parents
HOW TO SPOT IF YOUR TEENAGER IS ON DRUGS

In this day and age, it is easy to worry about whether your teenager is taking drugs.

The simple answer is yes, he/she is. But if you want to be sure, here are a few simple signs to watch out for.

DOES YOUR TEENAGER:

- Have regular mood swings?
- Go out with friends in the evenings?
- Sleep in late in the mornings?

IS YOUR TEENAGER:

- Prone to occasional spots around the face?
- Growing body hair?
- Bored with homework and showing an interest in the opposite sex?

If the answer to any of these questions is YES, they are on drugs. Confront your child.

Accuse them of being 'wide-eyed' and 'off the rails'.

Also go through their room, sniffing their curtains and identifying anything of ethnic extraction as a 'bong'.

They're bound to respect you more for it in the long run.

It does help to 'know the lingo'. Here are some alternative words your child may use when they actually mean drugs:

Heroin: horse, brown, bongo, H from Steps, 'nice one', 'safe', 'sorted'.

Cocaine: Charlie, barley, coke, blow, Rio, Coca-Cola, shouting powder, seafood chowder.

Speed: Monkey dust, Billy Whizz, sherbert, sugar, Sprite.

Ecstasy: Pills, bishis, E's, Westlife, Dr. Who, su-doku, video messaging.

Marijuana: Dope, blow (again), grass, pot, pook, tango, weed, reefer, hash, mash, cash, mobile, hoodie.

If you hear your teenager using any of these words, sending a friend a 'text', going to the 'cashpoint' or popping out for some 'chips'... well, you know what to do.

Ground them, call their head teacher and confiscate their mobile before they use it to go out 'happy slapping' or whatever.

The simple fact that the symptoms of being on drugs and the symptoms of puberty are almost identical should not distract you from the truth:

if you have children, they ARE going to take drugs.

Be grateful they're not off doing something worse, like 'daisy-chaining' or going to church.

Encourage your child to take their drugs where you can watch over them, like the living room or kitchen table; alternatively, encourage a hobby, such as watching TV.

Soon they will grow up to be just like you – tired, disillusioned, overweight and stuck in a job they despise – and you'll wonder why you ever worried about them.

These are NOT drugs!

COFFEE AND ALCOHOL

> 'People say alcohol is a drug,' snaps the comedian Chris Morris. 'It's not a drug, it's a drink.'

The same simple rule of thumb applies to coffee AND alcohol. If you ever worry that you might be becoming substance-dependant, look what you have in your hand.

If you can drink it, you're in the clear.

Having any kind of drink is socially acceptable, and as such neither harmful nor addictive. Anyone who tells you otherwise is at best an idiot, and at worst a student.

Sure, these products may contain active chemical ingredients, which can promote anti-social behaviour in the case of alcohol, or symptoms similar to cocaine in coffee (staying up all night, shaking, laxative release).

But the simple fact is that these substances are available in shops, or in service stations for bored motorists, and as such cannot be classified as 'drugs'.

Ask any scientist or politician and they'll agree.

Importantly, this does not mean these products cannot be treated the way you might treat a drug.

Vodka can be snorted (try it, it's wild). Instant coffee beans can be 'dabbed' onto a licked finger if,

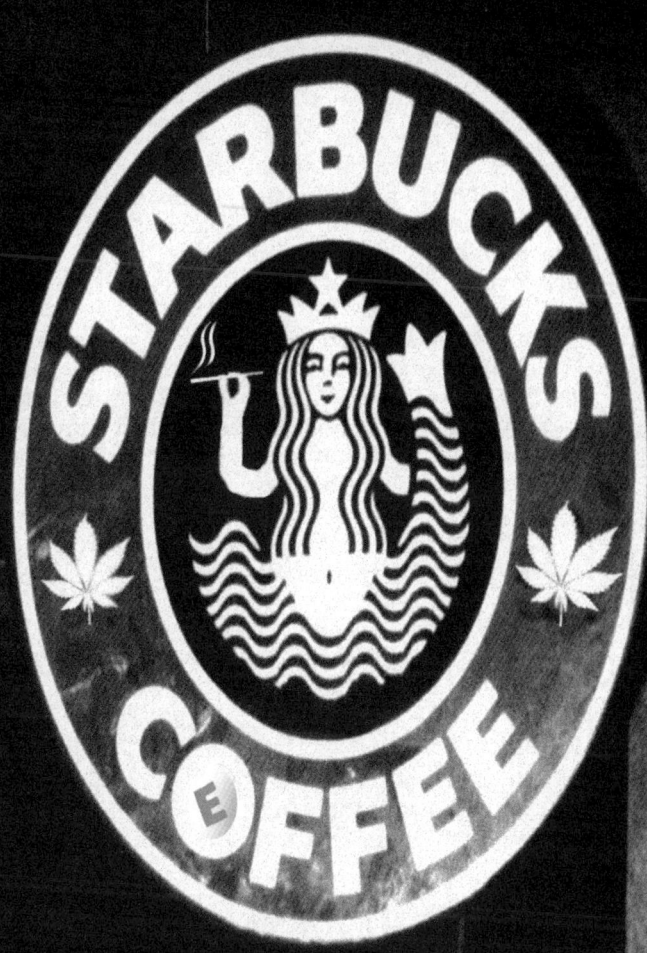

say, you need to keep yourself awake but have broken the kettle (the taste is repulsive, but then who ever chewed an E for the flavour?).

They can even be mixed irresponsibly (as in, 'Maybe just an Irish Coffee for the road'). Above all, either can become an addictive habit, part of your daily bodily cravings and – like any true drug – alcohol at least is best enjoyed in debilitating doses.

But don't ever kid yourself that you're taking actual drugs so long as you're doing anything you could happily do in front of your parents. And if you have the kind of parents who encourage you to skin up after dinner, or wink and nudge about you and your friends going off for a cheeky line, then find new ones.

> They have COMPLETELY missed the point of why you started taking drugs.

On the other hand, if your parents are alcoholics, remember they are only doing what society expects of them.

'MEDICAL' DRUGS

Ah, that old paradox – drugs designed to restore normality, rather than fuck with it. But let's not confuse prescription drugs with over-the-counter stuff.

Anything you can purchase without looking furtively over your shoulder is NOT a drug, as established above.

> It is, at best, a medicine.

> **Sure, you can nail whole bottles of cough syrup, it's a bit of a laugh when the drink runs out. Nurofen Plus hits the spot – it actually has codeine in it, which is why they keep it on the top shelf.**

> **Taking a bunch of Pro-Plus and then running round the neighbourhood – well, that's a spot of harmless ASBO fun for after homework.**

And if you want a challenge, try racking up and snorting a whole line of Lemsip – it's genuinely hard.

This is about as high as you can get in Boots.

But so long as you're not honest-to-goodness ill, illicitly-obtained prescription drugs cross the line from healthcare to joyride. They can range from blackmarket Viagra (see Sex and Drugs), via jellies (ask your corrupt local GP) to methadone (see Heroin).

Not all of them are this much fun, admittedly, but at least
– and this is key –
THEY DO HAVE THE BENEFIT OF BEING ILLEGAL.

DRIED-OUT BANANA SKINS

'They call it mellow yellow,' sang Donovan. They called him the 'Irish Dylan' – with good reason.

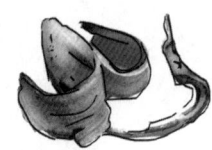

GLUE

This helpful little substance is primarily formulated for the affixation of two tensile surfaces. It is not intended for daubing into a Tesco bag before sticking your head inside (see diagram, How To Stick A Plastic Bag On Your Head). This is also true for other practical solvents, such as Tipp-Ex, Brasso, aerosols and magic markers.

Such products are actually more fun to use for their intended purpose, such as type correction, polishing and defacing private property. Even Amyl Nitrate is a safer and more pleasant way of obtaining a headache.

Still, if you ever feel your face is lacking for a few spots and sores, glue's your thing. Just make sure you don't attach your nose to anything embarrassing.

(I dispensed with the drawing of how to stick a plastic bag on your head because children may read this book and try it out.)

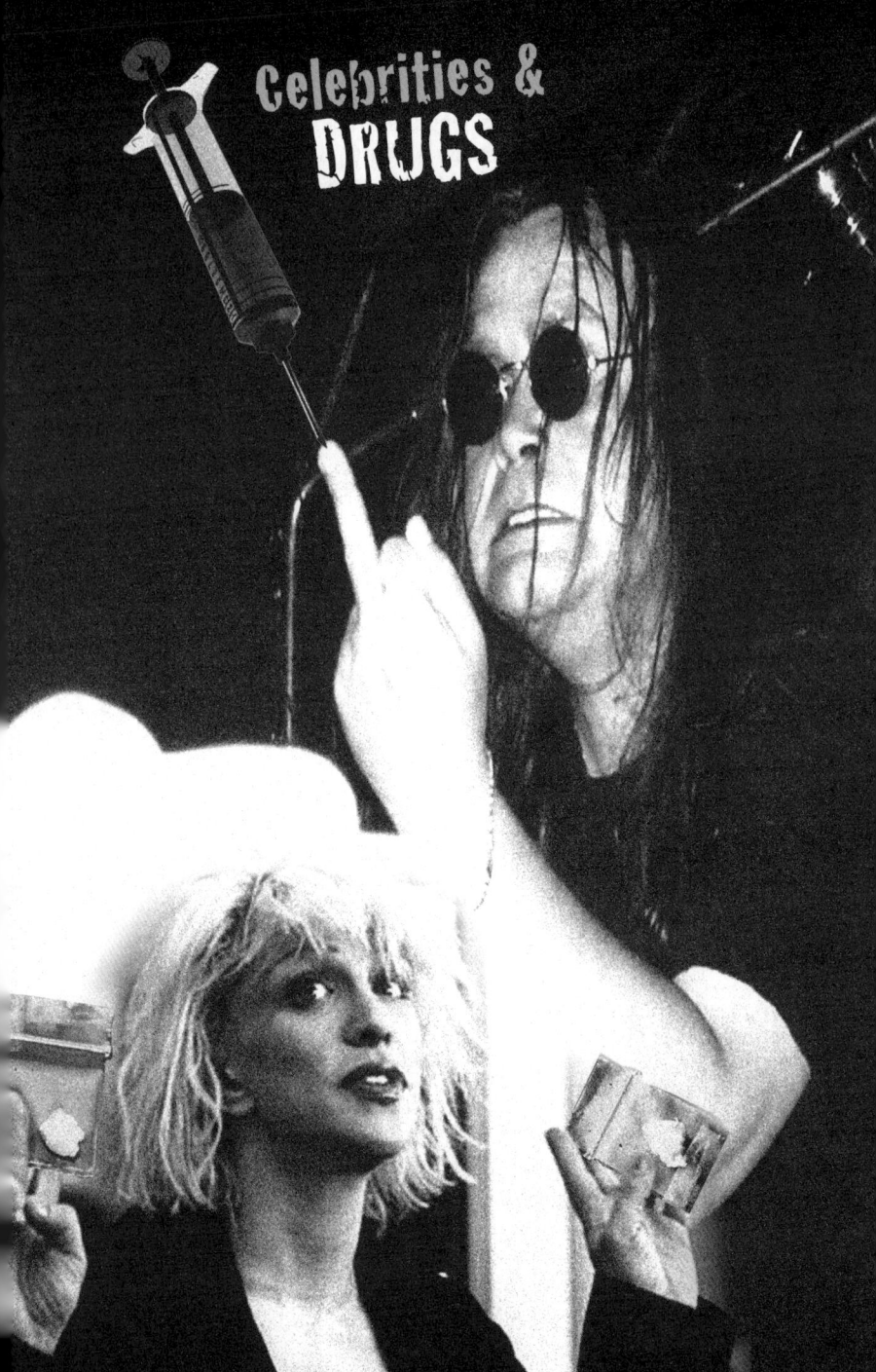

It is a well-known fact that ALL celebrities take drugs.

Many are paid directly in drugs for tax purposes. Still more have to smoke or inject moments before appearing on stage/ in parliament or they simply cannot perform.

However, the choice of drugs among the famous can vary widely. For example: Prince William will probably not have inherited the well-documented coke habits of his close relatives (eg Diana or James Hewitt). The standard experience of the user – that of believing oneself to be king, and having all the girls laugh at your every word – would be no different to how he feels when he wakes up every morning.

Well-known users:

Prince Harry **(pot, crack)**
Taki Takapopulous **(cocaine, amyl nitrate)**
Sid Vicious **(speed, heroin)**
Michael Barrymore **(ecstasy, aftershock, Viagra)**
Ozzy, Sharon, Jack & Kelly Osbourne **(all of them)**

Secret users:

John & Pauline Prescott **(Viagra, lots of, and blindfolds)**
Trevor McDonald **(coconut oil)**
Jonny Wilkinson **(kickamine)**
Charlotte Church **(nurofen, aspirin, money)**
Prince William **(speed, crystal meth)**

*Editor's Note: all the celebrities listed and their legal teams have fully concurred with our allegations. However, some names may have been changed and some facts made up.

All sources reliable and sober at time of research (about 3am during a lock-in).

Drugs and ANIMALS...

It has long been considered funny by students and delinquent teenagers to see how animals, especially beloved pets of other people, respond to drugs.

A psychologist would say they were exercising an atavistic right to assert man's power over beast, conducting a primitive act of revenge for the demeaned and animalistic state they themselves sink to when under the influence.

A sociologist would say they were little cunts.

Either way, cats on speed are considered the height of wit in some circles. Dogs vomiting up hash brownies, then spending an evening desperately frightened or confused, can also be very entertaining to certain individuals.

This author has only witnessed these events by accident, or in a controlled scientific environment, and has taken hardly any guilty pleasure from the observation. Some would argue that people who allow their dogs – or children – to truffle up human drugs like viagra, valium or ecstasy from their living-room carpet are not responsible enough to own a pet (or reproduce). I agree.

After all, what would people say if humans were to start hoovering medication designed for horses? *(See **Ketamine; fun with**)*

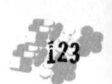

Drugs and TAXES...

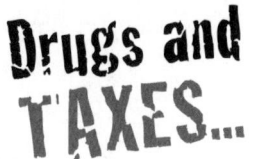

Remember: Always ask your dealer for a receipt. If possible get him to sign or initial it. Some may be reluctant to oblige but it is a little-known fact that small drug purchases are tax-deductable.

Buying off a street dealer has counted as a charitable donation since 1987. Back then a Conservative Future think-tank concluded that, since any money doled out to the homeless or ethnic minority groups only ended up in the drugs cycle anyway, there was no practical difference between subbing a beggar or buying the drugs yourself.

This scheme was designed to discourage the whole 'cash in hand' policy favoured by most pushers and purchasers.

NB: 1. Most pushers will ONLY accept cheques with a valid bankers card or blunt instrument.

2. Attempts to make card purchases WILL result in being marched to a cashpoint and forced to reveal your PIN.

3. Dealers make it policy to bring formal prosecution against any punter who attempts to skank them, however small the amount.

Finally, for amnesty on larger purchases the Inland Revenue will accept receipts and invoices whether in printed form, on headed cartel note-paper, or hastily scrawled on the back of a fag packet. The taxman isn't fussy about how he gets his slice.

TOP TIP: An added advantage of this good practice is that you will be able to return any suspect goods to the dealer and demand a full refund, or tokens to the value of the original purchase (participating dealers only)

DRUG TALK
Suggested topics of conversation...

In the rush to order the evening's drugs in, it is often easy to forget that you will end up having to talk shit all night. To many this comes naturally, but for others the inability to wax lyrical about geopolitics, personal morality and time travel can be an acute cause of social embarrassment.

PERHAPS you feel a bit uncomfortable lecturing strangers about social ills or how you'd run the country having just spent some people's weekly wage on 2g of pure shit. Not to worry, this in itself is a valid conversational starter.

POINT OUT CHIRPILY that one's easy relationship with your jovial West-End dealer must sit at odds with how he treats the penniless junkies on the street who don't pay up.

PERHAPS YOU CAN quote statistics to illustrate how many gang-related deaths in UK cities could be linked to the drug trade. Observe that, for your pleasure, only two or three links down the chain people probably died in Columbia or somewhere like that.

THIS WILL GIVE everyone something to nod sagely about before snapping up that next tempting line. It may even establish you as the 'really deep guy' everyone needs to have at drugs parties.

LIGHTER TOPICS of conversation include 'seriously scary' conspiracy theories, life on

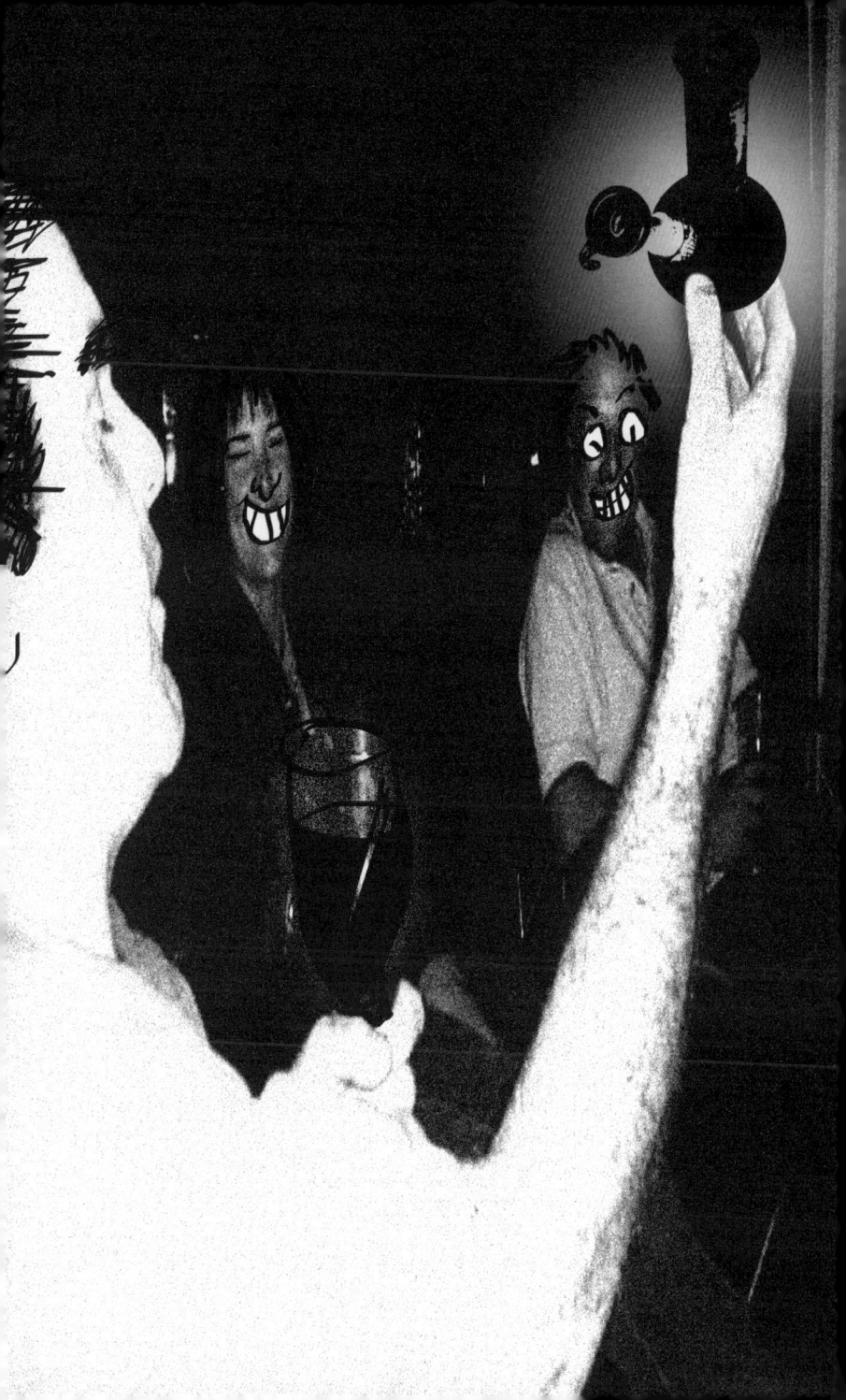

other planets and amusing porn footage 'some guy' bluetoothed you in the tube.

EARLY IN THE EVENING, keep it simple and the chuckles will flow; say, movies or TV shows which you and your friends can all quote from ('Did you see that bit where...'). This will persuade everyone they're in for a riotous evening of easy laughs, and relax them into ordering some more. Then, as dawn approaches, make sure you steer the chat towards something very important that you know absolutely nothing about (say, 'the paradoxes at the heart of Islam').

DO NOT ATTEMPT to discuss everyday banalities, like money or how depressing **Eastenders** is. This will disappoint anyone who didn't want to spend all that money on drugs to talk about something they discuss in a fag break at work, or overhear in a laundrette. And it's a fast-track to getting severely paranoid.

DO PLAN AHEAD. Ways to make yourself popular include stowing secret 'extras' to produce suddenly at 4am: perhaps a fresh 20 of Malboro Lights (cocaine) or a multipack of Mint Clubs or Penguins (marijuana).

Ultimately how much you enjoy your chat will depend on whom you choose to sail with that evening. Pick either trusted friends or total strangers: both are interesting in different ways, more importantly what YOU say will be – respectively – **either forgiven or forgotten**.

This is the final rogue's resort, the social climber's last foothold.

How to do DRUGS WITHOUT PAYING for them

If you're a woman, it's easy.
Coke for grope: you sleep with someone, they give you drugs and let you onto their yacht. You accompany them to the toilets, and they get to feel your tits. If you're really clever, you keep them going all night on the mere promise of sex without actually having to put out. The inevitable gets harder to put off the longer the evening wears on (you both get increasingly desperate for different things); but with a bit of luck he gradually becomes incapable and you slip off into the night with your consciousness heightened and your conscience virgo intacta.

With men, you have fewer natural bargaining chips.
Your ass will be good for a few pills in certain parts of town, but depending on your preferences this may seem like a higher price to pay than a few quid. Your best bet is to learn the twin evils of drug abuse: (i) the 'lost wrap' routine, and (ii) the 'lost tenner' routine.

Both involve making friends with more money than you; both involve potentially losing them. Round about 1am someone often claims to have 'lost' a crucial back-up wrap, and makes a big show of turning out their pockets.

Make sure to cling on to this guy: sure as hell he's gonna suddenly 'rediscover' it at 6am when hopefully it's just the two of you, claiming some kind of miracle. As for the other one... well, if you're the host for the evening, watch the scraggly gypsy guy in the corner like a hawk. And keep an even closer eye on your rolled-up note before it disappears into someone's pocket.

If you resort to pocketing someone else's tooter before the night is out, you thoroughly deserve the Hepatitis C you risk picking up from the bloodied end. It may cover your investment but you can't claim a victimless crime, especially not with a table full of people you know (or at least pretend to). Shame on you, as you hug the victim and tell him he's your best friend just half an hour later.

Essentially, though, drugs are like all luxuries... free to those who can afford them. **However, some people with too much money like to give it away to charity in order to feel better about themselves. So, you need to make yourself a charity case. Drug-addled trendies like nothing better than to support hangers-on who make themselves feel superior. Infiltrate yacht parties, aftershows, backstage and VIP areas... wherever the trendy rich gather to play. And you get free junk out of it, so everyone's happy. You may feel a small twinge within you – that's your pride hurting – but one of the functions of drugs is to anaesthetise moral pain.**

But (to paraphrase Oscar Wilde) when you're living beyond your means, sooner or later you'll be dying beyond them too. Not that you'll care so much then.

AFTERTHOUGHT: How to get out

So, decided you've had enough, have you? Well done, that's the important first step. Sadly it's also much the easiest. Actually giving up is a whole lot harder. It's not just the comedowns and the shakes. It's the realisation that the rest of your life won't be nearly as much fun that makes cold turkey look like, well, a slightly disappointing Boxing Day lunch.

So do yourself a favour. **This isn't a self-help book, there are plenty of those to waste your money on.** This is a self-harm book, pure and simple, and if you need reminding why, go back to page one and start again.

Better still, buy a new copy and read that.